21st Century
Pain Relief

21st Century
Pain Relief

Your Medical Breakthrough from
Chronic Pain to Vibrant Health

by Dr. Phillip Yoo D.C.

Foreword by Nelson Marquina, Ph.D.

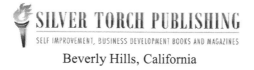

SILVER TORCH PUBLISHING
SELF IMPROVEMENT, BUSINESS DEVELOPMENT BOOKS AND MAGAZINES
Beverly Hills, California

21st Century Pain Relief: Your Medical Breakthrough from Chronic Pain to Vibrant Health

Copyright © 2013 by Dr. Phillip Yoo D.C.
www.lasermedinstitute.com
dryoo@lasermedinstitute.com

Silver Torch Publishing
www.SilverTorchPublishing.com

Library of Congress Control Number 2013935510
ISBN 978-0-9857581-3-4

Cover and back design by Carli Smith.
Edited by Gwendolyn Weiler

Printed in the United States of America.

This book is dedicated to my wonderful parents,
Pil Sang Yoo, M.D., and Mary Yoo,
who were always there to support me and my studies.

Table of Contents

Foreword

I was involved with developing the world's most innovative satellite-based imaging system when I was a Senior Scientist at NASA/Johnson Space Center. I also had the honor of being part of Ronald Reagan's "Star Wars" Strategic Defense Initiative using advanced multi-sensor imaging systems, high-power laser-based systems, and artificial intelligence.

As time went on, it was discovered that lasers have a healing effect on animals, and they have become widely used in the veterinary and equestrian industries. Since horses are fairly large animals, high-power lasers had to be developed in order to penetrate the deep tissues. Today, lasers have been successfully and safely used on humans. Popular examples are LASIK surgery for the eyes, certain dental procedures, disc nucleoplasty, skin care, varicose vein treatment, wound care, and many others.

I eventually discovered that certain lasers may be used to not only eliminate acute and chronic pain in humans, but also to regenerate damaged discs, bones, joints, and nerves; and heal soft tissue injuries. Furthermore, in all my years of extensive research, there is very strong evidence that certain lasers can stimulate some stem cells in damaged tissue and also favorably alter RNA synthesis and gene expression.

I have founded my own laser company in order to develop the world's most powerful lasers to heal the most challenging human ailments. Ironically, the ancients used light medicine to heal a multitude of diseases, and laser light is truly the future of medicine available today.

I may have developed the world's most powerful lasers, but Dr. Yoo is the one in the trenches of innovating the most effective ways of using the lasers to treat the worst chronic pain and nerve disorders encountered. I had the pleasure of spending time sitting with him in his backyard one day, listening to his big dream of reducing or eliminating the use of harmful drugs, risky injections, and unnecessary surgeries while using non-invasive laser medicine instead.

The biggest diseases in the U.S. are diabetes, cardiovascular disease, and cancer; we could list chronic pain as the fourth "disease". These conditions are all life-style related, and our national health care system should be focused on educating patients on the preventative benefits of proper diet, exercise, and, yes, getting enough light in their lives.

There are very few doctors who practice what they preach. Dr. Yoo not only talks the talk, but walks the walk by leading a healthy lifestyle himself as the founder of the Lasermed Pain Institute and being a bodybuilder, CrossFit instructor, and a teacher to his patients. He not only gets them out of pain, but shows them how to stay out of it by maintaining a healthy active lifestyle. (Yes, "Doctor" means "Teacher" in Greek.)

I hope that you will enjoy reading and practicing the recommendations that Dr. Yoo has for you in this book as much as I have.

Nelson Marquina, DC, PhD
Former Senior Scientist at NASA/Johnson Space Center
Former Manager, Advanced Technology Laboratories, GE
USA Laser Biotech Inc., CEO

Acknowledgements

I want to thank Dr. Scott Gillman, Dr. Bruce Coren, and Dr. Don Barry, who introduced me to cold and high-powered laser therapy. I would also like to thank Dr. Nelson Marquina who opened my eyes to the benefits of high-powered Class IV super-pulsed cold laser therapy as well. Furthermore, I am very grateful to have met Dr. Frank Jarrell, who introduced me to the Spinal Reflex Analysis (SRA) infrared thermo scanner and technique, which allows me to diagnose and treat with pinpoint "laser" accuracy. These doctors have all showed me the healing power of light.

I am also grateful for all the instructors of the International Federation of Sports Chiropractic (FICS), especially Dr. Greg Uchaz, Dr. Tom Hyde, Dr. Brian Nook, and Dr. Jay Greenstein. These doctors are on the forefront of developing the most innovative sports chiropractic techniques, and all their hard work and dedication has allowed our profession to officially be a part of the Olympic Games, as well as other professional sporting events worldwide.

I would like to thank all the trainers at CrossFit Football for getting me back into shape, especially 10-year NFL Veteran John Welbourn, whose groundbreaking knowledge of correct technique in exercise, sports performance, and proper diet will transform the athletes of the future.

I extend thanks to Icon Builder Media, especially David and Jill Fagan, and Gwendolyn Weiler, for helping me with creating, editing, and publishing my first book.

I also would like to thank all the military, special forces, and veterans who I have treated, as they have put themselves in harm's way so that you and I can live in a free country.

A special thanks to the members of the Christian Chiropractic Association, especially Dr. Bruce Kniegge and Dr. William Hollensed, who supported my mission trip to Central America.

I would like to thank my clinic staff - Lauren, Tina, Angie, and others - who have delivered the most high-quality and compassionate health care to all my patients.

A special thanks to my wife Angela, and kids, David and Kathy, for putting up with me all those late nights and weekends where I sacrificed valuable family time to further my laser studies and finish this book.

Another huge thanks to all the brothers at the International Church of Christ, especially Pastor Jaeho Park, Jaeden Park, Kevin Springer, and Andreas King, for keeping me in alignment spiritually.

Lastly, my greatest appreciation goes to God, the creator of life-giving light, and my Lord and Savior, Jesus Christ, who was the ultimate healer.

Part I
In The Beginning

And God said, "Let there be light," and there was light. God saw that the light was good, and he separated the light from the darkness.

- Genesis 1:3-4

Chapter 1

Meet the Doctor

*"Night pierces my bones; my gnawing **pains** never rest."*

- Job 30:17

Pain.

You are reading this book because you want to get out of it.

I've spent my whole life creating it, seeking it, enjoying it.

As a serious bodybuilder, Spartan Race competitor, and CrossFit trainer, I have studied all the intricate details of pain. I push until my strength dissolves, and then I put in a mile more, or push through that extra rep of squats, deadlifts, pull-ups, or presses. It is there, at the frayed end of my performance, that I have drunk deeply of pain; even reveled in it.

When my body is pulsing in unison to the throb following my workout, I know it was enough. The soreness that cradles me the next morning brings a smile to my face because I know that I went the distance.

But the twist in this story is that after it has played its part, I need to put it away and move on. So I can do it again.

In my professional life, this means I make an incredible doctor. As it says in Proverbs:

"Do you see a man skilled in his work? He will serve before kings; he will not serve before obscure men."

- Proverbs 22:29

I have traveled the world studying the most effective traditional and non-traditional methods of pain management. After a 16-year sojourn treating everyone from top military officials, elite special operations units, and ambassadors from every continent; Olympic, NFL, & Major League Baseball Athletes; top entertainers, and even other medical doctors in pain, I have put together the ultimate non-surgical, non-needle, non-drug pain elimination protocols using the future of non-invasive laser medicine.

Furthermore, my unquenchable thirst for more knowledge, more treatment techniques, more innovations, and more improvement in my skills has forced me to forevermore add to my arsenal of the latest and greatest treatment modalities.

You are reading this book because you want to be out of pain. I am writing it because I offer something that may be able to help you – without the use of dangerous drugs, invasive injections, or severing surgeries. In the future, man will look back and be bewildered by the medieval, butcher-like surgical procedures we use today, which have failed to manage chronic pain and have often caused more harm than good. As good old Star Trek Doctor Bones McCoy of the U.S.S. Enterprise would say, "Dammit Jim, I'm a Doctor…not a Butcher!" (The good doctor used non-invasive lasers and energy to heal his patients.)

My goal goes far beyond wanting to get you out of pain fast. I am also someone that is striving to give you your life back, your body back, and your hope back. As you will see throughout the coming pages, I will never ask you to just take my word for it. I will share with you countless clinical case studies and patient testimonials, including my own, that will help give you a thorough tour of what I've already been able to do for top athletes, elite soldiers, entertainers, your neighbors, and other people that are suffering from the same things that you are.

But it's also important to me that you understand where *I* have been. I am not just your treating physician – someone who is working with "Star Trek" technology to help relieve you of pain. I am also someone just like you. I have struggled with debilitating pain that threatened to shut down my life, and I, too, was in search of a solution. So it is also as your peer – not just your doctor – that I share with you my own story.

My Story

My experience with pain has not all been well. After graduating from Michigan State University with a degree in health education and human performance (yes, I am a Spartan; Aroo!), I became a personal trainer. I walked the walk and talked the talk, maintaining my own rigorous training program. One day, I was doing a deadlift – a power-lifting movement where you lift a heavy weight off the floor. It was something I'd done hundreds of times before. But this time, something went wrong and I was in immediate pain.

Normally, if my back got a twinge, it would just go away. But not this time. The pain did not subside, and it got continually worse. I soon realized I had seriously injured my back.

As a personal trainer, I recognized that my career was on the line. As a human being, I saw that my quality of life was on the line. For any of you who have suffered from relentless back pain, I don't need to tell you how crippling it can be.

I ended up going to see a chiropractor. I was amazed by the results. I was not only out of pain, but my performance ability increased. He left me better than he found me! That was truly a blessing in disguise, and a life-changing experience for me. I became really passionate about this magic called chiropractic. I went back to finish pre-med school and became a chiropractic doctor myself.

The Journey Begins

Right after graduation, as a practicing physician, I went on a mission trip to Honduras in Central America. I'd originally only intended to be there for one month, but tragedy set a different plan in motion.

Another doctor picked me up from the airport when I first arrived in Honduras. We were car-jacked on the way back to his home, and he was shot in the eye. After getting him to the hospital, I decided to stay in the country and take over the medical mission on his behalf. For the next year, I lived and worked in a country where there weren't more than a handful of chiropractors.

I served and treated hundreds of patients. This was different than what I'd seen back home in the States. I wasn't working with upper-middle class Americans coming in for their weekly visit on their way to the salon or professional jobs. I was dealing with farmers and field laborers who had nothing but their own two hands and a strong back for making a living. I was handling the worst cases there, and the consequences of our success or our mishaps were grave.

I didn't just rely on chiropractic; I took on the perspective of a whole-body doctor. What worked? What didn't? Being in a third world country, there were no regulations restricting my scope of practice. And because there was a lack of primary care physicians in the mission field, I had to fulfill that role as well. I used all available resources: pain medications, parasite medications, chiropractic, Chinese medicine, you name it. If the therapy existed, I was willing to try it. In fact, that's where I was first trained on, and experimented with, prolotherapy injections. I trained under a local Honduran medical doctor on how to combine prolotherapy with acupuncture, and got amazing results.

I was driven to understand the causes of back, joint, and other pains and how to cure them.

A Pioneer in Korea

After a year, I took my curiosity and ambition to Korea, where I was the first American-born chiropractor to serve the U.S. Army, Air Force, and Special Forces personnel serving in Korea. I worked with other doctors to spread my knowledge and passion for this non-invasive science. My heavy client base was mostly made up of expatriates, active duty military, and military contractors. I also had the honor of treating Korean actors such as Lee Byung-Hun (who starred in the movie *G.I. Joe*), the Korean National Track Team, and ambassadors from four different continents, just to name a few.

Below are three classified military documents and letters of recommendation from the highest-ranking military officials. The first is from the Brigadier General from the Special Operations Command Korea; the second is another classified letter of recommendation from an Army Colonel in charge of the dental clinic, one of the doctors I treated during that time. The third document is a certificate of appreciation signed by the United Nations Combined Forces Command, United States Forces-Korea 4 Star General Deputy Commanders.

As I treated these military personnel, it occurred to me again that these were individuals whose daily sustenance depended on their ability to walk out of my office in good condition. I continued to search for better ways to solve the problems in front of me. I began to experiment with Eastern medicine, and eventually married it with the Western therapies I'd learned back home.

Testimonial 1

UNITED STATES FORCES KOREA
SPECIAL OPERATIONS COMMAND KOREA
UNIT #15622
APO AP 96205-5622

REPLY TO
ATTENTION OF

SOJ0   5 July 2009

MEMORANDUM FOR To Whom It May Concern

SUBJECT: Letter of Recommendation for Dr. Phillip B. Yoo

1. Dr. Phillip Yoo has been treating Special Operations Command Korea (SOCKOR) personnel for over a year now and comes highly recommended. His thorough understanding of the daily rigors that the members of SOCKOR endure and the extra time he takes to study the mechanics of each soldier's injury enhances his ability to fix the root cause of the condition for long term relief.

2. I started seeing Dr. Yoo myself for chronic neck pain I'd been experiencing since May and have gotten excellent results. Before seeing Dr. Yoo, I had difficulty turning my neck all the way, but after just a few of Dr. Yoo's treatments I feel much improvement. As a pilot, it is imperative that I maintain full range of motion in my neck in order not to impede my visibility and performance while flying. And as a General, it is important that I maintain good posture to present an authoritative image as well as set a good example to those under my command. Dr. Yoo has educated me on proper ergonomics and exercise in order to do just that.

3. Furthermore, Dr. Yoo has volunteered his time by offering to come to the gym on post and conduct some cross-fit training classes, in which he is a certified instructor. Therefore, I can only say that Dr. Yoo has shown a total commitment to provide excellent care and service to my special forces personnel here at USFK, and I am confident that he will do the same wherever he goes.

Sincerely,

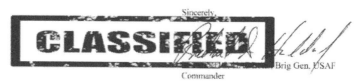

Brig Gen, USAF
Commander

Testimonial 2

DEPARTMENT OF THE ARMY
US ARMY DENTAL CLINIC
FOX ARMY HEALTH CENTER
REDSTONE ARSENAL, AL 35809-7000

REPLY TO
ATTENTION OF

MCDS-SECR   15 October 2009

MEMORANDUM FOR RECORD

SUBJECT: Recommendation for Dr. Phillip Yoo

1. I strongly recommend Dr. Phillip Yoo for the selection MD-DH-10-8406, chiropractor.

2. Dr. Phillip Yoo was my chiropractor during my last six months while I was stationed in the Republic of Korea. He came very highly recommended by many active duty as well as civilian personnel. I had suffered from severe back pain and immobility for over a year and a half due to multiple herniated discs. I had exhausted all the treatments available through our military medical system in Korea with no relief. Dr. Yoo put me at ease immediately with his gentle and professional manner. He is extremely skilled and knowledgeable. I followed his treatment plan which included an exercise rehabilitation therapist and within less than a month, I no longer needed any analgesics; my mobility was greatly improved and I my whole outlook had improved.

3. As a care provider myself, I encountered many active duty patients in the Korea that suffered from painful musculoskeletal conditions. I recommended Dr. Phillip Yoo to each and every one of them. I personally met with my Brigade Commander in Yongsan to bring to his attention the tremendous need for a chiropractor, Dr Yoo in particular, for our Soldiers in Korea.

4. All patients that I had sent to Dr. Phillip Yoo returned to me to thank me for the recommendation. Dr. Yoo speaks Spanish and Korean fluently. In the past he has enthusiastically supported health fairs and in-services at the Brian Allgood Hospital at Yongsan by volunteering his time and expertise. Dr. Yoo's friendly and caring manner, work ethic and professionalism will be a true asset to the military health system. He should be selected for this position without reservation.

5. Point of contact for this memorandum is the undersigned at ████████████; cell ████████████ email: Robin.

CLASSIFIED DOCUMENT

COL, DC
Officer-In-Charge

Testimonial 3

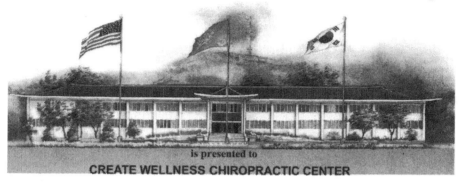

United Nations Command
Combined Forces Command
United States Forces Korea

CERTIFICATE OF APPRECIATION

is presented to

CREATE WELLNESS CHIROPRACTIC CENTER

In appreciation for your unselfish and untiring efforts in ensuring the success of the 6th Annual ROK-US Combined Forces Command "White House" Holiday Party. Without your tremendous contributions, this remarkable endeavor would not have been possible. Your dedication and support serves as an inspiration and symbolizes the strength of our great ROK-US Alliance. Kamsa Hamnida – Katchi Kapshida.

SUNG CHOOL LEE
General, ROK Army
Deputy Commander

December 15, 2008

WALTER L. SHARP
General, United States Army
Commander

The Olympics in Beijing

My next stop was China, where I was invited and credentialed to treat Olympic athletes participating in the 2008 Olympic Games held in Beijing. Talk about pressure! I had just one or two chances to get these Olympians back into their competitions. It was an honor to be able to meet and treat current athletes as well as retired legends like the World Olympians Association President Dick Fosbury, who invented the "Fosbury Flop" high jump technique and won the Gold Medal in Mexico in 1968.

I teamed up with other sports doctors and we continued to combine Eastern and Western medical procedures for great results. It was here that I was first exposed to laser therapy and how fast it worked on the athletes. We were a revolving door of miracle-like cases.

Backstage With Beyoncé

After establishing my reputation for being able to get top pro athletes and military personnel back to their peaks as soon as possible following debilitating injuries, I caught the eye of multiple entertainers. I had only been back in the United States for a few weeks before I received an email asking if I would treat the Beyoncé crew and staff during her tour in Seoul, Korea.

This wasn't the first time I was asked to treat a world famous musician. A few months earlier, I had been asked to treat the Pussy Cat Dolls at their hotel. I didn't take advantage of the opportunity at the time because they weren't able to come to my clinic, where I had access to the best equipment which would have provided them with the best care. Besides, it was a Friday night at the end of a long week, and I was eager to get home and spend time with my wife and kids, so that's what I did.

But the next day, I felt guilty as I read in the paper that two of the Dolls were unable to perform due to severe back and knee pain. I had refused to use my God-given treatment skills to get these girls functional and back on stage. I was determined not to make the same mistake again.

When I was asked to be the backstage therapist for the Beyoncé tour, I didn't hesitate to take the offer. At first, I mostly treated the sound and stage crew for lower back pains and the drummer, who was suffering from tight shoulders. But as my reputation spread, it wasn't long before I was treating more prominent members of the entourage. One of Beyoncé's main backup dancers complained of a misaligned hip; then came the production manager, and even the head of security.

Treating the head of security was the key to getting unlimited access and the best view in the concert hall, which was the side of the stage where you could see everything up close without anyone blocking your view. I ended up going back and forth between my treatment area and the concert without any hassle from security officials, as I was now their new friend.

From the audience and fans' perspective, we only see what goes on onstage and don't realize what these performers and backstage crew put their bodies through while touring around the world. I, for one, can appreciate more what these entertainers and staff members go through, and I know firsthand that singing and dancing is not "easy money." Your body pays the price.

The Lingering Perspective

My time abroad was critical to my life's purpose. I was so fulfilled getting farmers back into the fields, soldiers back on their missions, athletes back into the game, and entertainers back on stage. I served such a wide spectrum of individuals, each of which represented such extreme medical cases. These were people that needed me; and not just for minor improvements to their everyday life, but for enabling them to *sustain* their lives.

This put the necessary pressure on my performance to encourage me to go that extra mile, even after the pain and exhaustion had set in. Just as I would push myself in the gym during my own training, I had to put my game face on and continue to search and seek and research and serve. In the end, my research spanned across several years and four continents. I thought I'd tried it all.

As happy as I was to have built up such a well-stocked toolbox of modalities and therapies I could use, I came face to face with this stark reality: I didn't have a magic button. All of the therapies I'd been using had limitations: drugs, physical therapy, surgery, injections, steroids – even chiropractic, my first love. There were lots of failed cases with each of these procedures.

I came to the conclusion that although the combination of allopathic and alternative therapies benefited most of the population, there were always those stubborn cases that did not respond to the tools I had to offer. But I also believed that there was something more I could do – something else out there I had not yet discovered – that could help relieve the pain of even the most unyielding cases.

Finding the Answer

Back in the States, the answer came disguised as yet another injury. I hurt my back during vigorous CrossFit exercises. At first, I thought I'd just pulled a hamstring; but a medical evaluation concluded with a diagnosis of spinal disc damage and sciatica. It sounded grim.

In addition, I had been suffering from severe peripheral neuropathic pain in my back, buttocks, leg, and groin – a curse from a bad case of the shingles. To add insult to injury, I had also developed some idiopathic neuropathic numbness, tingling, and pin-like sensations in my lateral foot and ankle. Furthermore, I had developed a type of compression injury in the gym, causing numbness and pins and needle-like sensations in my right forefinger, especially when typing.

I was a mess. But I wasn't too worried. Unlike the first time I'd been crippled by an injury, now I had a whole spectrum of solutions to my physical problems. Or so I thought.

I soon realized that nothing was working. *I* was proving to be one of those infamous stubborn cases. Honestly, that was a little awkward, since I was supposed to be the rainmaker when it came to relieving pain. Yet there I was, helpless to help myself. I couldn't even drive more than 30 minutes without my pain reaching a 10 out of 10, with knife-life pain shooting down the back of my leg. The only things I didn't try were highly potent pain killers, epidural injections, and surgery – all of which I never even considered as options due to their risky side effects.

So I did what I'd always done. I kept looking for answers. And I found one.

I met Dr. Nelson Marquina, Ph.D. He was a senior NASA scientist who had worked on Ronald Reagan's "Star Wars" Strategic Defense Initiative, where he helped design high-powered lasers to shoot down any nuclear missiles threatening to invade U.S. airspace. Dr. Marquina had since switched his focus to medical lasers and introduced me to the world's most powerful 60-watt Class IV high-powered laser, which I currently use in my own practice. After less than a month of therapies, my debilitating pain went away. I went back to living an active, pain free lifestyle.

In fact, I had yet again been left better than I had been found. The laser therapy gave me relief from my entire list of ailments and even gave me super hero-like powers. Okay, maybe I couldn't shoot lasers from my eyes like superman, but it's true that I was able to break my own personal record and do 20 nonstop repetitions of barbell squats, bearing more than one-and-a-half times my body weight (270 pounds), without any support belt or shoes. Mind you, this was performed within just a few short weeks *after* being diagnosed with the slipped disc and receiving the laser treatments. (You can see this incredible feat by typing in "Dr. Phillip Yoo Squats" in the YouTube search bar.) Furthermore, around the same time, I was able to deadlift 405 pounds, again without any support belt or shoes.

As far as I was concerned, I'd just discovered the Holy Grail of non-invasive pain management. I figure that if I, at more than 40 years of age, could lift tons of weight off the floor after surviving a prolapsed disc, then I should be able to get many of you disc sufferers out of pain, and able to lift up your golf clubs, laundry baskets, or even your 50-pound grand kids!

I was infused with passion. Just as I had devoted myself to the science and procedures of chiropractic after witnessing firsthand what it could do for people, I knew that I needed to learn more about the laser therapy and adopt it as part of my practice. In all of my searching and studying, it was a hole I hadn't been able to fill before. But now I had it – the answer.

The laser helped me all those years ago, and it's something I still go to as my first line of defense for my own physical problems. I have had a total of four different experiences with neuropathy – all of which have been successfully treated with the laser technology. As much as I suffered during those times, there's a sense of satisfaction that comes from being able to be my own success story. I can tell you that I have seen countless patients with my own eyes get out of ridiculous pain after suffering for a long time and trying every treatment and specialist in the book. I can cite peer reviewed literature, clinical case studies, scientific formulas, and even throw in a few patient testimonials; but at the end of the day, I can tell you without a doubt that it works because it has worked on me - multiple times.

Now, I want to share that with you – as literally and figuratively as possible. What I want to extend to you in the following pages is some background information about what it is we offer at the Lasermed Pain Institute in Newport Beach (Costa Mesa), California, and how it may be able to change your life. Just as my doctors have consistently left me better than they found me, I aim to do the same for you.

But you don't have to take my word for it. We'll let my patients and their results speak for themselves.

Chapter 2

The Problem of Pain

*"Light in a messenger's eyes brings joy to the heart,
and good news gives health to the bones."*

-Proverbs 15:30

Pain dulls the senses and casts a shadow across the rest of your life. The things you once found fulfilling or important now stand downstage as you measure your life in minutes and hours. This could be the bite of physical pain as you suffer through a sports injury, severe back pain, or the aftermath of surgery. Or, it could be the emotional trauma of watching your ability to live your life slowly disappear as you struggle against neuropathy and other nerve disorders that chip away at your ability to use your body to its fullest extent.

Whatever your personal situation might be, you know first-hand what it's like to have your priorities dramatically rearranged as a result of an unwanted physical condition. Where you once had vitality and strength, now you are left discouraged and desperate. You can see how it's affecting your daily life, and how it affects the people around you. Spouses and caretakers worry over your wellbeing, and your relationships may be stressed as a result.

You may have a limited ability to work and make a living. Even if you are able to be there in person, your performance may be suffering as your mind is constantly being pulled back to your physical situation.

If you're a pro athlete or weekend warrior, you may be experiencing the fear of an early retirement, or having to give up the sport or exercise you love. You may be distracted by the uncertainty of how that will affect the rest of your life as you become less active, leading to undesirable weight gain and loss of strength, muscle mass, and vitality. You may be thinking about how this forced sedentary lifestyle also increases the risk of the three big killers: Diabetes, Heart Disease, and Cancer.

If you're an actor, entertainer, or model, you may be unable to perform at your peak due to work-related repetitive stress injuries, not to mention the stress on the body from all the long days on sets and having to constantly travel around the world.

If you're in a Special Forces unit in the military, active duty, or a veteran, you may have injuries sustained while being deployed on a combat mission, or just physical wear and tear from the years of repetitive stress on your body, caused by carrying a heavy backpack and gear while marching and training for days and years on end. It is needless to say that military hospitals and clinics are poorly equipped and understaffed. This results in you not getting the proper pain care you need. This only causes the condition to get worse, often requiring the once active-duty soldier to get a boring desk job that won't strain damaged discs, muscles, and joints.

You may have been medically discharged because your pain has progressed to the point where it disables you, and you have to face the fear and uncertainty of losing your career. You recognize what this means — that in addition to the personal way it affects your life, the thousands of dollars and hours the government spent training you to do a job you can no longer perform (and the thousands more it will pay in your disability benefits, if you are one of the lucky veterans to get through the red tape) is a loss to your entire community. You may fear that you will be left with only a broken body riddled with chronic pain.

If you're a baby boomer or senior, you may be wondering if you're on a downward slope that will never end, and fret the day you will have to give up the car keys, hang up the golf clubs, and be sentenced to spending your remaining years pent up in a nursing home, confined to a wheel chair because you let your health deteriorate into permanent disability.

If you're a mother, you may be feeling guilty over the loss of your ability to meet the physical needs of your family, whether it is picking up the kids from school or soccer practice, or simply going grocery shopping and making a nice dinner.

If you're a health care practitioner, you may be struggling with the irony of working to cure others' maladies while you are unable to treat your own.

Here is how some of our patients described their suffering:

The pain was so bad day and night I hoped it did not have to eventually come to them amputating my feet. I have taken all sorts of medication you can think of, and nothing worked… I went to another doctor and it did not do me any good; I still had the pain day and night.

- **Dr. Joseph F. Cavon, M.D.,** Mission Viejo, CA (see the full testimonial on page 92

I have had severe pain from neuropathy for the last 20 years, -and crippling for the last year - that caused me to lose my balance. I have no feeling in my feet that goes up the anterior portion of my leg. I have been to my primary care physician who has prescribed me with pain medication and referred me to a podiatrist who put me on Lyrica and Cymbalta without any effect. I was also referred to a neurologist that put me on Gabapentin.

- **Carla Visnic, RN,** Anaheim, CA (see the full testimonial on page 24)

I came in with a protruding L4 and L5 lumbar. Basically, it is the worst pain I have ever experienced. I play volleyball for my college and this pain began in April of last year. I really did not think much of it. So around that June I started to seek help from different doctors and chiropractors. The doctors told me to do stretches and pain relieving exercises, but nothing was helping me.

- **Harley Frost,** San Juan Capistrano, CA (see the full testimonial on page 62)

I had herniated discs and a shoulder that ripped. I had to have surgery. At first my spine did not bother me, but as time passed, it started to give me this excruciating pain. All the doctors I saw only prescribed pain medications. It was like they were taking my wounds and wrapping them in bandages.

- **Nettie Gonzales,** Los Angeles, CA (see the full testimonial on page 65)

Does that sound familiar? Could you paint an even more dramatic picture of what you're going through on a daily basis?

Either way, I'm sure you'll agree that there is no story more relevant to your life than your own. That is why you may not be as interested in the problems presented in this book as you are the solutions that offer hope.

The Things We Do For Relief

At this point, you may feel that you have tried it all. As someone who is suffering, you have searched, read, dug, and searched some more. There is probably not a stone you have left unturned. It always follows the same pattern: you yearn for relief and then someone tells you about something that you haven't tried before. Is it herbs? Chiropractic? A wonder drug? It doesn't matter. It's something that you have not tried — something that has not yet failed — and so it embodies hope. It is a possibility.

You hungrily delve into this new possibility. You undergo the treatment, you spend the money, and you cross your fingers.

But then it doesn't work. It's another dead end. And now you have the added discouragement of the possibility that *you cannot be helped.* You are living with the fear that this may be it – this may actually be as good as it gets - and you will have to live this way forever. Or worse, your situation is continuing to grow in severity and urgency, and it's like watching a train coming towards you at full steam. You can do nothing but watch the closing distance between you and that unstoppable force.

But wait! A friend, a magazine, or a doctor tells you about yet another solution – something else to add to the till of possibilities. Do you dare to hope? Of course you do. What else is there to do? So you try, try, and try again.

And so the cycle goes.

It's nice to be unique, but in this situation you loathe being the exception to the rules. The therapies, medications, and other modalities that have helped others have left you in a pool of disappointment and throbbing pain. Your physical situation is a stubborn case that refuses to yield to the things that *should* work. These are things that perhaps have worked for you in the past, or things that you have witnessed work for others. So, why not you? Or why not this time? Why are you consigned to a constant state of static improvement?

You know first-hand that the only thing more discouraging than your daily struggle is the hopelessness of not knowing how to stop it.

Surgery: Why or Why Not?

As someone that has been the victim of excruciating, ongoing pain I understand the desperate measures that we are willing to go to for relief. But for me, I never even considered surgery as an option.

Doctors will sometimes recommend surgery once they feel a patient has exhausted all other options, but this is a rough way to go. Sure, they have arthroscopic methods that are less invasive than a scalpel. But you still need to take the small, but potential risk of going under anesthesia, and have them go inside your body and cut, slice, and stitch…or whatever other invasive procedures they need to do.

For example, when you have vertebrae that have thinned out and begun to put pressure on your nerve, this can be very painful and lead to other medical issues. In the case of surgery you will be opened up, the disc material will be physically removed, and then replaced with a spacer. But there is additional hardware required in order to hold the artificial disc in place. This usually consists of two rods being secured along the spine with four titanium screws. But it's after you've been stitched up and sent home that the real problems begin.

For one thing, the hardware comes loose 80% of the time. This can put pressure on the surrounding area and cause things like permanent nerve damage or infection. The other problem is that, even if the procedure is successful, it is meant to fuse your moving parts together;

it's working against your body's natural design. The vertebrae above or below the fixed joints will now have to bear the burden of the static vertebrae, which eventually leads to the deterioration of those areas, too. This then leads to additional surgeries of the same exact nature. It's a snowball effect. Not to mention that these kinds of procedures can cost up to $169,000.

Even if your insurance covers the cost of the procedure, there are other costs involved. You may have to miss extensive time from work in order to recover. This is not only true for the initial surgery, but since there is such a high rate of further damage, it is more than likely that you will have to take additional time off in the future. And if the procedure fails to be effective, then you are overall in much worse shape than you were before. Now you've missed work, undergone the physical trauma of major surgery, and your body is housing foreign hardware that may cause further damage.

Obviously, surgery is not the best choice, and should be avoided if at all possible.

But *can* it be avoided? As we mentioned at the beginning of this section, surgery is what doctors recommend after they feel all other avenues have been exhausted. So what else is there besides surgery that offers that last hope for relief?

This would be a good time to tell you that these hopeless cases are my specialty. They have been my passion for years. It's not enough for me to be able to solve the problems for the majority – I need to know how I can help the few. I have been there. I know the scary, desperate place that you've found yourself in, and I know it is ugly.

But I also know the relief that has come through finally, *finally* finding the solution. In the next chapter, I hope to bring you to the end of your long, exhausting journey to find relief.

Chapter 3

The Search is Over

"The doctor of the future will give no medicine, but will instruct his patient in the care of the human frame, in diet and in the cause and prevention of disease."

- Thomas Edison, 1847-1931

My patients' health concerns range from arthritis, fibromyalgia, and neuropathy to sports injuries, bulging, herniated, degenerated discs, and sciatica. When they come to the Lasermed Pain Institute, they are searching for real pain relief after conventional medicine has failed to help them. Often, they've been recommended to undergo high-risk invasive surgeries, epidural injections, or prescribed medications, such as non-steroidal anti-inflammatory drugs and opiates that temporarily mask pain, but are rife with dangerous side effects. Instead of relying on these modalities, I recommend high-intensity laser therapy as a first-line treatment for anyone suffering with acute or chronic pain.

As mentioned in the first chapter, I discovered this treatment, my own Holy Grail, after a long, exhausting search that spread over several years and four continents. It wasn't until I was looking for relief from my own debilitating pain that it manifested itself. I was fortunate to discover the Class IV high-powered laser, as shared by Dr. Nelson Marquina, Ph.D., which became the crowning jewel in the comprehensive treatment plan I offer my patients.

Today, I am the only one in the entire country utilizing *both* the world's most powerful, FDA cleared safe, 60-watt Hot Laser, and the 250-watt super-pulsed cold laser. This means that even if you have tried some kind of laser therapy before, you haven't tried these.

What Makes Our Laser Different Than Others?

The ability of a laser to deliver sufficient photonic energy in deep tissue is proportionate to the laser's power, which is measured in watts. Most Class IV lasers only produce six to 15 watts of photonic energy. However, our lasers are the highest powered lasers in the world and deliver a whopping 60-250 watts of continuous - or super-pulsed - photonic energy, and are thus five to 33 times more powerful than any other laser out there.

The diagram below shows how our highest-powered lasers in the world are able to penetrate deeper into the body's tissues, which results in more efficient, faster, and effective treatment outcomes compared to all other Class IV, and less powerful, cold lasers.

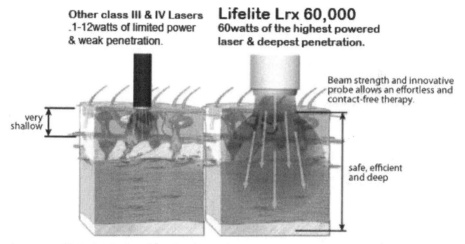

Other class III & IV Lasers .1-12watts of limited power & weak penetration.

Lifelite Lrx 60,000
60watts of the highest powered laser & deepest penetration.

Beam strength and innovative probe allows an effortless and contact-free therapy.

very shallow

safe, efficient and deep

Lasermed Pain Institute Is The Only Lrx 60K Laser Provider On The Entire West Coast!

I have three different laser units with different characteristics. I select the one (or the combination of the three) best suited for a health problem after a thorough review of the medical history and unique pain issues.

Each disease benefits from a different laser. Generally, I use the hi-powered Class IV 60-watt hot laser for muscle, bone, joint, and disc diseases; the hi-powered infrared health light therapy for peripheral neuropathy and chronic pain; and the hi-powered Class IV 250-watt super-pulsed cold laser for the healing and regeneration of stem cells, organs, connective tissues, and the outer coverings of nerve tissues (the myelin sheath). These different lasers may or may not be combined with each other and techniques such as electrical therapy, clinical nutrition, or other modalities mentioned later in this chapter.

As you can see, my collection of lasers, as well as the other methods unique to my practice, enables me to treat all aspects of the human body. My comprehensive treatment plan has been referred to as legendary, but I like to think of it more as futuristic. It's something you would expect to see on Star Trek. Today, I offer you full access to this cutting edge, comprehensive approach to your pain relief.

How Laser Therapy Works

The lasers I use have a fiber optic cable that connects the laser machines to a Star Wars light saber-looking handheld device the size of a flashlight. The laser is placed directly over the injured area for several minutes, depending on the size of the area being treated and the dose provided by the laser unit.

Studies have shown that when tissue cultures are irradiated by lasers, enzymes within the cells absorb energy from laser light. Visible (red) light and Near Infrared (NIR) light are absorbed within the mitochondria and the cell membrane. This produces higher ATP levels and boosts DNA production, leading to an increase in cellular health and energy. The process can be compared to photosynthesis in plants – sunlight is absorbed by plants, which is then converted to usable energy so that the plant can grow. There is strong evidence that the laser energy stimulates stem cell regeneration and favorable DNA and RNA gene expression in damaged disc, nerve, and joint tissue.

When human cells absorb this light-energy, it initiates a series of

events in the cell that eventually result in normalizing damaged or injured tissue by stem cell stimulation. This stimulates nerve regeneration, muscle relaxation, and immune system response and reduces pain, inflammation, edema, and the overall healing time by increasing intracellular metabolism – a process called photobiostimulation ("photo-bio-stimulation"). Lasers have no effect on normal tissues, as photons of light are only absorbed and utilized by the cells that need them.

All light is composed of photons. Photons are small packets of light energy – in the form of waves – with a defined wavelength and frequency. Photon energy is able to more effectively penetrate the skin and underlying structures, therefore accelerating the healing process. Light travels at a constant speed and oscillates up and down as it moves forward. However, all light is not the same. It is measured in wavelengths, with each wavelength of light representing a different color of the spectrum. The number of oscillations per second represents the frequency of each wavelength; shorter waves have a greater frequency than longer waves. Laser energy is coherent (well-ordered photons), monochromatic (single-color) light energy. When produced as a narrow, bright beam, laser light holds its intensity until it is absorbed by a medium (the body). When applied to an organism, laser light, tuned to specific wavelengths and frequencies, stimulates metabolic processes at the cellular level.

Summary of the Photochemical Process:

Photons

Absorbed in Mitochondria and Cell Membrane
within cytochromes and porphyrins

Singlet Oxygen is Produced

Changes in Membrane Permeability

ATP Synthesized and DNA Produced

Increase in Cell Metabolism from a
Depressed Rate to a Normal Level

Selective Bio-Stimulatory Effect on Impaired Cells
(Note: cells and tissues functioning normally are not affected)

PHOTO-CHEMICAL EFFECTS	PHOTO-MECHANICAL EFFECTS	PHOTO-THERMAL EFFECTS
The cell equilibrium, altered by the pathologic process, is restored. Inflammation is reduced and the analgesic response is very fast.	Pressure waves stimulate the lymph draining system in deep layers. The rapid resorption of inflammation mediators and leaked liquids is achieved.	Circulation is stimulated so more oxygen and nutrients can reach the suffering structures.

Can It Work For You?

Whether you are suffering from a chronic or acute ailment, you are a candidate for this process. It works, regardless of your malady, because it is working with the body's natural healing process to promote your speedy recovery. It is not like a drug or therapy that targets just one area of the body and cannot cross over to your other physical needs, or creates side effects for other systems.

However, the healing properties manifest themselves differently for different things. For instance, if you're struggling with neuropathy, your body is going through a different healing process than it would be for something like degenerative disc disease. The therapy itself is not introducing – or inducing – anything into your body that was not already there. Instead, it is giving your body more juice so that it can use its own devices to recover.

Three Case Studies:
NFL Pro Athlete, Registered Nurse, and Neighbor

Below, I will introduce to you to three different people with three different medical issues – all of whom found relief through my proprietary Lifelite Laser Protocols. You will see that I do not offer a cookie-cutter solution for cookie-cutter issues. I treat a wide range of issues, and I am confident that you may also find relief with my proprietary Lifelite Laser Protocols, too.

Case Study #1:
NFL Player, David Jones (DJ)
Bulging Disc with Sciatica

Pro athletes push their bodies to the max. It is no wonder that there are often injuries that need to be dealt with. My experience working in the 2008 Olympic Games has given me a unique edge when treating other serious athletes. I realize that a quick recovery is essential in order to get my patients back in their game as soon as possible, and as safely as possible.

NFL Player David Jones (also known as DJ), former Offensive Tackle for the Baltimore Ravens and Philadelphia Eagles, came to my office with a bulging disc, a bad case of sciatica, and damaged ankles and feet – obviously all football injuries. His medical issues were the result of years of repetitive, heavy physical trauma from playing football since he was in elementary school. This was not his first time being in pain, but he wanted it to be his last.

"When I was in the NFL, I was getting anti-inflammatory pills, which didn't do much for my situation with my back and disc. The team athletic trainers and doctors did not do much for me. So I flew all the way from the East Coast to see Dr. Yoo in California. I've been coming to Dr. Yoo for about three months, three times a week now, and I can actually feel a significant difference in the way I feel. For instance, I've been sitting down in my car and I haven't been able to feel the pain shooting down from my sciatic nerve as much anymore. I know when I first came to see Dr. Yoo, my pain was usually about an eight, and now after these treatments, I can honestly say I've been around a one or a two on a pain scale of 10. I can now sit down for longer periods of time without it hurting. Dr. Phil also made some custom-made sports orthotics for my flat feet, which have put my whole body back in balance, and now I can walk and run pain free! Now I have the option of getting back on the field, as my agent is getting offers

from several teams. If you have any problems that are similar or equal to mine, I would suggest you come to Dr. Phillip Yoo, because I definitely believe that this laser therapy works."

(You can see DJ's live video testimonial by typing "DJ Jones Laser" in the YouTube.com search bar.)

Case Study #2:
Registered Nurse Carla Visnic
Diabetic Peripheral Neuropathy, 20 years

Medical practitioners spend a lot of time on their feet. They work late hours, and their health lends itself to the professional care and healing of their patients. When a practitioner is in pain, or is not able to satisfy the demands of his or her job, it causes a ripple effect. I feel that ensuring their health and well-being is a service I perform not only for them and their families, but for the people they serve.

Registered Nurse Carla Visnic came to my office suffering from crippling neuropathy. It all started with some numbness and tingling in her toes that her family doctor said was from wearing her shoes too tight. This kept gradually increasing over the years until her feet felt like they were filled with Novocain or wrapped in bubble wrap, and felt too heavy for her to carry.

"I have been a nurse for 40 years and work on my feet a lot. I have had severe pain from neuropathy for the last twenty years, and crippling pain for the last year that caused me to lose my balance. I have no feeling in my feet that goes up the anterior portion of my leg."

At night, even just the weight of her bed sheet felt too heavy, too hot – a burning she couldn't get away from. Walking around on the cold kitchen tile helped a little, but she was losing a lot of sleep every night. At work, she was noticing her balance was getting worse. Her neurologist drugged her up with maximum doses of Gabapentin, Lyrica and Cymbalta. These drugs made her feel like she was "out of her mind." She was told that there was no cure for neuropathy and that pain management by drugs could make her life livable.

Her pain and numbness increased even under all the drugs and was getting so bad that she was increasingly unsure about her footing. Carla and her family began to seriously worry about her falling and really hurting herself.

Every day, Carla and her family's life centered on dealing with her neuropathy; it had taken over her life. With tears in her eyes, she told us that she was beginning to really wonder how long she could go on living this way.

"Then one day, I was researching through the Internet and came across Dr. Yoo's site. I came to his clinic, and after just three clinical trials my pain went from a 10 to a six. I have feeling in my feet now after so many years. I am also able to do things that I have not been able to do in years, like exercising! The tingling feeling is almost completely gone and I just feel like a miracle has occurred."

(You can view Carla's amazing transformation by typing in "Carla Neuropathy" in the YouTube.com search bar.)

Case Study #3:
Cheryl Michaels
Disability Eliminated and Mobility
Restored after Multiple Car Accidents

Whether you're an entertainer, an athlete, a veteran, or a medical professional, pain is an inevitable part of life. When that pain comes, it's important for you to understand what your options are so that you can resolve the issue, then go on with your life. You are someone's neighbor, friend, family member – *your* life has a ripple effect. Getting out of pain means getting you back into your life, and back into the life of your loved ones.

Cheryl Michaels of Costa Mesa, CA, came to my office with limited mobility after she'd been in multiple car accidents. Her life revolved around seeking relief for her condition. She'd tried everything, with little to no success. She described her transformation during treatment as a miracle. These are her words:

"I was a victim of car accidents. I literally could not walk. I was in and out of the hospital getting shots in my back. I went through chiropractic. I went through acupressure, which did help a little bit to relieve pain. I was told I was going to be crippled in four years. I tried everything – pain management, everything. I went online and found Dr. Phillip and after the third laser treatment, I am able to get out of my bed; I can walk up and down stairs; I don't wake up in

excruciating pain, and I'm sleeping better. It's a miracle. It's a miracle."

(You can see Cheryl's incredible transformation by typing "Cheryl fibromyalgia laser" into the YouTube.com search bar.)

This isn't magic – This is science

Albert Einstein – not George Lucas – was the first person to imagine laser technology, which he referred to as "stimulated emission." As early as 1917, he understood that each color of light represents a different frequency – a different wavelength. The colors we see are a compilation of the different lights being emitted from atoms when they are struck by light.

Einstein theorized that he could create a mass emission of the same wavelength of light by using mirrors to reflect the atoms' light right back into it. The back and forth reflection of the light would build until it would finally trigger a massive chain reaction of light – a laser beam.

As ground breaking as the theory was, it proved to be too mature for its time. It wasn't until after World War II that this science was seriously revisited. The first laser wasn't even invented until 1960. From there, many prototypes followed. Scientists were astonished to discover that therapeutic doses of laser light could stimulate the body's healing processes. They could mimic some of the sun's attributes, and actually benefit the human body. This started a flood of research. Papers were published and it was a race to see who could find the ultimate panacea first.

Today, lasers are widely used throughout the field of medicine. The Class IV hi-powered laser stands at the evolutionary peak of this technology. The key is in the body's absorption of the laser light energy. As it sinks into the skin and subcutaneous tissue, the body's healing mechanisms are stimulated. The longer the wavelength, and the higher the power output of the laser, the deeper the photons can penetrate into the body.

There are several models circulating the market right now that are too weak to provide the kind of healing I'm talking about. Low-level laser therapy requires extended treatment times in order to even come close to rivaling the healing outcomes of the highest-powered 60-250 watt Class IV lasers in the world. And I'm sure you'll agree that when it comes to pain, the faster you can get out of it, the better.

Successful Clinical Case Studies

"After one laser treatment, I have not had any pain."

Morton's Neuroma

"I read about Dr. Yoo's laser treatments in the L.A. Times. I suffer from Morton's Neuroma and have had pain in my feet 24hrs a day 7 days a week for 20-plus years. I have been to a neurologist, podiatrist, deep tissue massage therapy, and reflexology. I would not take any medicine, so the pain level for me was always high. After one laser treatment, I have not had any pain. In the 20-some plus years when I ran and hiked mountain trails I used to have pain, but now I no longer have that pain. So thanks Dr. Yoo."

Kathy Adams, Palm Springs, CA

(You can see Kathy's raving review by typing "Kathy's neuroma laser" into the YouTube.com search bar."

"Despite my Parkinson's, I can walk with a normal stride without having to shuffle my feet."

Parkinson's Tremor & Numbness from Cancer Medications

"Hi, I'm Bob Schellenberg. I'm a former catcher for the Philadelphia Phillies organization. I met Dr. Phillip Yoo two weeks ago. I came into meet him, after having his laser therapy services recommended to me by a friend. I gave him my health history, which included having a deep vein thrombosis several years ago due to a senior league baseball injury, which developed a blood clot and went to my lungs. I had a bilateral pulmonary embolism... A few years ago, I was diagnosed with parotid gland cancer behind my right ear which caused a few problems. The most aggressive of those symptoms is early onset Parkinson's. I have a tremor in my right hand, which was confirmed a couple of weeks ago as definitely Parkinson's. I was having some shuffling sensation in my right foot, and after six treatments with Dr. Yoo's laser, I've been able to walk with a normal gait, with less sensitivity in my feet, less neuropathy, and with less tingling and numbness

sensations in my feet. I still have the tremor, and we're hopeful of addressing that as we move forward, but so far I've been delighted with the results we're getting with the laser.

Bob Schellenberg, Huntington Beach, CA

(Check out Bob's miraculous transformation by typing in "Bob, Phillies Laser" into the YouTube.com search bar.)

Chapter 4

A Comprehensive Approach to Healing

"Their fruit will serve for food and their leaves for healing."

- Ezekiel 47:12

As I mentioned in the first chapter, there are many other treatments out there that have a high success rate, but still have a margin of failure. You may have found this to be true in your own life, as you have tried things that have worked well for others around you. Perhaps these are things that have even worked for you in the past. I had that experience myself, so I can understand that frustration first-hand.

However, I have found that when these options are combined with the laser therapy, they are worth trying again. The Lifelite Laser Healing System is a unique protocol designed to provide rapid relief from pain. When you come to my clinic for care, you will find a thorough treatment plan to address your unique health issues. Although the laser therapy is my first line of action when a patient comes to me with pain, I also use other complementary treatments and modalities that help to accelerate your healing and make you more comfortable.

The Graston Technique with Laser Therapy

I am the only practitioner combining laser therapy with the Graston Technique®. This technique incorporates a patented form of instrument-assisted soft tissue mobilization, which was originally developed by athletes for the treatment of sports injuries. Today, more than 16,000 clinicians worldwide use this technique to treat acute and chronic soft tissue injuries. The technique is able to detect and effectively treat areas of the body suffering from soft tissue fibrosis (scarring) or chronic inflammation.

After an injury, the buildup of excessive scar tissue may limit your range of motion and cause pain. This can hinder your ability to resume life as normal and extend the trauma of the event that caused the injury, whether it was a sports injury, the aftermath of a surgery, or other injuries. The instruments used in the Graston Technique are concave and convex-shaped handheld stainless steel instruments, which the practitioner rubs against the problem area, using very specific methods, to help break down the scar tissue and promote a healing environment.

Using a cross-friction massage, which involves brushing or rubbing against the grain of the scar tissue, the practitioner re-introduces small amounts of trauma to the affected area. This temporarily causes inflammation in the area, which in turn increases the rate and amount of blood flow in and around the area. The theory is that this process helps initiate and promote the healing process of the affected soft tissues.

After the Graston treatment, the laser is then used to heal the area at a cellular level with photonic energy and increase the healing process a hundred fold. The Graston Technique offers relief, and combining it with high-powered laser therapy means relief comes even faster. In fact, I am currently using this technique on myself in order to treat carpal tunnel syndrome – something I picked up from my time in the gym. After combining the laser with the Graston Technique, I have now restored about 89% of the mobility back into my wrist, and expect more to follow.

I am currently working with an Aerospace Engineer to custom make a more ergonomic and improved set of tools to my exact specifications, as they will be designed to work in conjunction with the hi-powered laser therapy. (I will be training and certifying doctors on this innovative treatment modality called the "Laser Edge" Tools & Technique. If you are a doctor, you may find out when the next seminar will be by visiting www.lasermedinstitute.com.)

What the Graston Technique Does:

- Works the areas of tissue buildup in order to stretch and splay the connective tissue and muscle fibers. This separates and breaks down the collagen cross-links.
- Breaks down dysfunctional tissue and makes it more functional.
- Increases the circulation to the problem areas.
- Helps to relax chronically tight muscles.
- Increases the cellular activity in the treated area.
- Warms the treatment area so that the laser will be even more effective and the tissue will absorb more photonic energy.

Benefits of the Graston Technique with Laser Therapy:

- Decreases overall time of treatment.
- Allows patients to continue to work and maintain physical activity.
- Reduces or eliminates the need for splints, braces, and other physical assistants.
- Fosters faster rehabilitation and recovery of the injured area.
- Reduces or eliminates the need for anti-inflammatory drugs.
- Aids in the treatment of chronic conditions thought to be permanent.

Case Study: A Former Pro Volleyball Player's Tale

Dijon Douphner, who is a former U.S.A. Men's Team pro volleyball player living in Huntington Beach, CA, came to see me several years after a collapsed chair left him with painful bulging discs in his neck and back. Prior to the accident, he enjoyed an active, athletic lifestyle. He was anxious to find relief and go back to spending his afternoons outdoors. He finally came to my clinic for help after exhausting his options and trying many different therapies and drug options. He was at a point where he was taking a high volume of pain pills, but they didn't even work anymore.

When he first came in, I did the standard compression test, where I extend the head back a little and push down on the top of the head. Even that small amount of pressure I applied sent lightning bolts down his arm. An MRI confirmed there was a severely bulging disc in his neck. Honestly, I wasn't sure if I could help him; I wondered if he'd need to get surgery after all.

> *"When I came in initially, my range of motion was limited; anything that was beyond the plane of my body – if I were to tilt my head up even a few degrees – would be enough to send my arm shooting with numbness and tingling. I had almost a constant numbing sensation between my index finger and thumb. Any motion to the left and any extension would aggravate that and make my arm just go numb… I actually had to walk around all day, and sleep in such a way, that my head was constantly flexed because if I even brought it into the same plane, my arm would go numb."*

After three months of the laser decompression, we were both amazed by the results, and equally relieved that he was able to avoid surgery. When a disc bulges or herniates, the weakest area is the outer wall of the disc, which either cracks or fissures and allows the disc material to ooze out. When the laser delivers the photonic energy to the area, it's being absorbed by the damaged disc tissues. The laser heals the area, which is kind of like it's welding the cracks or fissures shut. This prevents the nuclear material from oozing out and pressing on the nerves. This not only relieves the symptoms, but goes to the root cause of the problem and corrects the issue for permanent results.

> *"Now I'm back to a regular posture, where I can keep my head up and I have full extension again."*

But there was a secondary issue; he also had a huge lump of contracting muscle and scar tissue clouding the top of his left shoulder, since the muscles were trying to compensate for the weakness of the disc.

> *"I had never had a lump or bulge or any type of deformity in the muscle prior to maybe six or seven months ago; then I noticed it in conjunction with my neck going awry – that I had this knot there. So when I came in, one of the techniques he was using was the Graston – you know, just running over it with the tools. I mean, [the knot] actually disappeared the quickest. Within a couple of months that had gone from a huge, literal bump that you could roll over, to being completely gone."*

What we did was use the Graston Technique to mechanically break up all the fascial adhesions by running over the area with a series of different smooth, stainless steel tools. This process also helped the disc to heal because it was bringing in the additional blood and circulation, and taking the inflammation out of the area. The rubbing warmed the treatment area so that the laser would be even more effective and the tissue would absorb more photonic energy.

(You can see the hi-powered laser in action as I worked on Dijon's discs by typing "Dijon's Disc Laser" into the YouTube.com search bar.)

Applicable Conditions:

The Graston Technique has been successfully used to treat the following:

- Cervical sprain/strain (neck pain)
- Carpal Tunnel Syndrome (wrist pain)
- Lateral Epicondylitis (tennis elbow)
- Rotator Cuff Tendinosis (shoulder pain)
- Achilles Tendinosis (ankle pain)
- Scar Tissue
- Shin Splints
- Lumbar sprain/strain (back pain)
- Plantar Fasciitis (foot pain)
- Medial Epicondylitis (golfer's elbow)
- Patellofemoral Disorders (knee pain)
- Fibromyalgia
- Trigger Finger

(See the Laser Graston Technique in action as it helps to alleviate shoulder pain in a pro athlete, prior to his winning a golf tournament where he averaged 290 fairway drives, by typing "Dr. Phil Yoo treating former AVP volleyball player" in the YouTube.com search bar.)

Spinal Decompression with Laser Therapy

After traveling the world and doing extensive research on the most effective, non-invasive method to treat pain caused by herniated, bulging, and degenerated discs I have invented the Lifelite Laser-Neuroflex Decompression Proprietary Protocols, which combine multiple non-invasive treatments, including Open Architecture Spinal

Decompression Therapy and the world's most powerful 60watt-250watt Class IV Laser Therapy, to treat chronic pain and inflammation caused from disc and nerve disorders. This unique combination of therapies helps to magnify the body's natural healing mechanisms and get the patient to a new level of comfort and wellness as fast as possible without having to resort to popping pills, poking needles, or painful surgeries.

What It Is

The KDT Neuroflex Spinal Decompression Therapy is a treatment that utilizes alternating traction and release forces in order to gently decompress the protruding discs. The patient lies on a decompression table on their back, stomach, or side-lying position while a special computer applies gradual levels of distraction to gently pull apart the spine, allowing the disc to reform to its proper shape. With some decompression machines, the doctor doesn't touch the patient at all. However, I often combine it with Leander Flexion Distraction, which is a hands-on approach where I apply pressure to the area, because I believe the combination adds another dimension to restoring the normal pump mechanism of the damaged discs.

What the machine does is gently pull the vertebrae apart, decompressing the pressure on the injured disc. Our unique KDT Neuroflex table also flexes the vertebrae, allowing further opening up of the disc space. This creates negative pressure so that the disc can go back to its correct space. This is done in a repetitive motion. With each repetition, joint fluid is pumping through the area and making it easier for the disc to go back between the vertebrae through a process called "imbibition." The mobility also trains the muscles around the area so they don't atrophy. This therapy accelerates the healing process by alleviating strain on the injured disc, while restoring its access to the body's natural flow of nutrients.

Coupling this procedure with the Class IV 60-watt Laser Therapy offers expedited pain relief and faster healing. Our technique, which we refer to as our proprietary open belt architecture decompression technique, allows us to administer the photonic energy while the client is on spinal decompression. The decompression opens the disc space so the laser can penetrate between the disc vertebrae as deeply as possible for maximum results.

With the vertebrae open, the photonic energy is able to thoroughly target the damaged part of the disc and nerve tissue and help the body to heal itself faster. As the photonic energy is able to penetrate deep into the area, the body produces increased amounts of ATP (Adenosine Tri-Phosphate), which is the substance responsible for cellular energy production. This natural process improves circulation, reduces painful inflammation, and allows the body to heal three to five times faster than it would otherwise.

Case Study: A Registered Nurse's Tale

Rose Gomsi, a registered nurse in Santa Ana, came to my office with neck pain, low back pain, and sciatica. As a medical practitioner, she is on her feet all day as she works to meet the needs of her patients. Here's what she had to say about her first visit:

"This morning I was a mess waking up. I had a stiff neck, which was like a number eight or number nine [on the pain scale]. And I came in here because after work I had hip pain earlier, too; so it was hip and neck. The hip pain had been an eight or nine, and when I came in here it was probably a seven or eight. And the neck was probably an eight. But after an hour, when I've had all the therapies and the decompressions, and the laser I can say my neck now is maybe a number three and my hip is a number three. I feel like a new person again. I could just go back home and have a nice dinner and not be in pain."

Rose continued her treatment after the first day, and here's her report after many more visits:

"After fifteen treatments of laser and decompression, my back pain is a zero, my neck pain is a two, and my sciatica is a zero. Now I am able to play tennis with no ill effects to my back or hip. I am really pleased with the treatment, and I am so excited that now when I get off work I can make dinner and enjoy it without any pain. Thank you so much, Dr. Yoo."

(To see Nurse Rose's testimonial, type "Rose Neck and Back Pain Testimonial" into the YouTube.com search bar.)

Spinal Reflex Therapy with Laser Therapy

I am currently pioneering another combination of therapies with Dr. Nelson Marquina, Ph.D., a former NASA senior scientist who worked on Ronald Reagan's "Star Wars" antimissile laser defense program. We are also collaborating with Dr. Frank Jarrell, the founder of the Spinal Reflex Analysis (SRA) Institute, in order to combine other state-of-the-art techniques with his SRA protocols. These protocols use an infrared laser thermo scanner so we can find, with pinpoint laser accuracy, the root causes of nerve dysfunction and chronic, unresolved pain syndromes. Therefore, this new protocol is like a GPS system that helps the practitioner navigate exactly where and how to treat a patient using Spinal Reflex Therapy with the hi-powered super-pulsed laser treatments.

What It Is

First, you need to understand what a spinal reflex is. It is a normal, defensive withdraw reflex in response to stimuli that you can neither see nor hear. For example, if someone creeps up behind you (unseen and unheard) and throws a glass of cold ice water on your back, the spinal reflex will induce you to instinctively jump up and turn around to see where the splash came from. Breaking this example down even further, the reflex is the automatic activation of a large number of muscles – without you even thinking about it. A moment later, after the reaction has occurred, your body will calm itself and go back to normal on its own.

The problem occurs when an injury or chronically unstable area of the body creates a spinal reflex to get stuck in the "on" switch. Instead of inducing a sudden contraction of muscles, then subsiding, the muscles stay contracted and excited. These muscles then put strains on the corresponding spinal joins, causing a compression on the associated nerves.

Spinal Reflex Therapy (SRT) begins with a Spinal Reflex Analysis, which enables the practitioner to identify the source of the on-going reflex causing trauma to the body. Once the problem area – the root of the problem – has been identified, the SRT calms the area and turns the reflex "off." This causes a domino effect throughout the body: the cessation of the reflex causes the muscles to relax, which relieves the

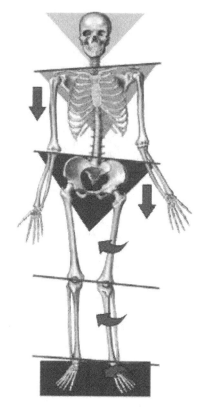

pressure on the spinal joints, which neutralizes the pressure on the nerves, etc.

Using the 45-watt to 250-watt hi-powered super-pulsed cold laser in conjunction with this technique will topple the dominos even faster. Residual areal tenderness will be reduced; the body will heal faster from the extended effects from the reflex; the injured area will repair itself faster with the blast of photonic energy, which will keep the problem from recurring again.

This is an exciting endeavor for us. As always, I am on the constant lookout for new and innovative ways I may be able to serve my patients with faster pain relief and healing.

The Foot Factor

I take a whole-body approach to your medical issues because I understand how each part of the body interconnects with so many other systems. One thing that many physicians overlook is how important your feet are to your overall health. Think about it – they are about 10 inches long, 4 inches wide, and support your entire weight all day, every day.

Luckily, the designer of your body recognized how important your feet are. A healthy foot acts as a spring and can easily bare the weight of your body. However, over time, as environmental factors take their toll, and as more and more people are plagued by obesity and other health issues, the foot loses the ability to act as a spring. For instance, in the case of obesity, the foot can roll in and the body's weight is being distributed to other areas of the foot it wasn't intended to be.

When your feet lose their springy characteristics, they no longer absorb the shock of your body. The shock of every step is being redistributed to other parts of the body and foot. The brunt of the labor is put on the discs and knees. With the constant pounding of your body (walking down stairs, walking from room to room, exercise, etc.), the discs and knees start to thin out, causing a wide array of physical issues.

The resulting fascia strain also creates other problems throughout the rest of the body. Fascia is the membrane coating all of your muscles – like Saran Wrap. If a muscle is damaged, it can cause the fascia to gather in on itself and clump together, pulling on the other connecting tissues. That means that pains manifesting themselves in certain parts of your body may actually be the result of fascia strain from another area. This is one of the many reasons we take a whole-body approach to your wellness.

We do a head-to-toe analysis of each patient. There are times that I will recommend custom-made orthotics that will restore the shock absorption in your foot area, and eliminate the fascia strain. This, in turn, eliminates pain in other areas and brings the upper body back into proper alignment. It's simply one more piece in the holistic approach to your care.

This is something that is both an aid for correcting structural problems in the body, and for avoiding problems in the future. You don't have to wait until your body is strained in order to consider this option. For instance, some minor league sports associations require orthotics for all of their players in order to keep injuries to a minimum. If you are an athlete, or someone that is putting a lot of strain on your body on a regular basis, this is something that we can use to give your body the extra support it needs.

Case Study:
Former Super Bowl Champions Baltimore Raven's NFL player DJ Jones' custom made orthotics

When former Baltimore Raven's player DJ Jones came to my office, he was seeking treatment for a bulging disc, a bad case of sciatica, and a damaged hamstring – football injuries that one may not immediately connect with the feet. His physical analysis, however, showed a perpetual weakness in his foot and ankle that was creating a fascia strain that was causing it to pull other things out of balance, too.

Creating his custom orthotics was an important part in his care, as it helped to maintain the benefits of the other therapies we were administering. Otherwise, that weakness would have continued to sabotage his treatment plan. The strain from that area would have still been pulling the other areas of his body out of balance, and prolonged his treatment program. The orthotic was something that supported him both off and on the field.

(To see our secret step-by-step process of how we provide the world's best foot assessment and orthotics casting process and products, which are the first choice among Pro Athletes, type "NFL Player's custom made sport orthotics" into the YouTube.com search bar.)

The Rebuilder Procedure

The Rebuilder Procedure is the use of a therapeutic device that produces electric current to stimulate the nerves to fire at a normal rate of 7.83 Hz. It opens up the nerve pathways, soothes irritated nerves, and wakes up numb nerves. The Rebuilder causes a very soothing sensation. The signal feels like a tiny tingle that pulses on and off. You can manually adjust the intensity setting for maximum comfort. These signals produce a gentle buzzing feeling. These tingling impulses then reverse direction and go from one foot all the way back to the other. In this way, all the nerves from the lumbar area down to your feet are treated.

Lifestyle Changes

There is only so much that I can do for you as your physician. I can be your mechanic, but you are the driver and owner of the vehicle and should take necessary precautions to ensure good health. This will go a long way in helping you avoid chronic diseases and illness, and it is also a good way to better manage existing health issues.

Things You Can Do

There are many things you can incorporate into your life, like better nutrition and exercise programs, which will go a long way in helping you find relief.

In addition to maintaining good habits, you may also need to focus on eliminating bad ones. For instance, smoking and excessive alcohol consumption undermines your body's healing mechanisms. Poor diets lead to nutritional deficiencies and weaken your body's natural defenses against disease.

- Maintain Optimal Weight

This can help to reduce the physical strain on your body and avoid weight-related diseases like Diabetes II. You can start the weight-loss process by keeping a food journal; trading processed foods for fruits, veggies, and whole grains; and starting an exercise program.

- Avoid Exposure to Toxins

In Southern California, we are surrounded by unwanted toxins, which can put additional strain on our bodies. That's why it's important to do what you can to avoid the ones you *do* have control over, like caffeine, alcohol, tobacco, pesticides, etc.

- Correcting Vitamin Deficiencies

Vitamin deficiencies can manifest themselves as a variety of painful, physical symptoms. You can determine whether you are lacking certain vitamins through a blood test, but you can also take proactive measures to address any possible deficiencies by taking a quality multi-vitamin. I can't emphasize "quality" enough, though. This industry is largely unregulated, so the best way to be sure you're taking something beneficial is to choose a distributor based on a referral from a qualified physician (like me!)

For patients suffering from neuropathy, I carry the Neuropathy Support Formula, which is a special combination of vitamins and minerals that have been backed by many clinical studies to show they help with Neuropathy symptoms. Some of these include: Vitamin B1 (Benfotiamine), Vitamin B2 (Riboflavin), Vitamin B6 (Pyridoxine HCI), Vitamin B12 (Methylcobalamin), R-Alpha Lipoic Acid, and Vitamin D, along with many other vitamins.

)

Chapter 5

Crossing the Bridge

*"Then your light will break forth like the dawn,
and your healing will quickly appear..."*

- Isaiah 58:8

Now is the time to decide your next move. Please understand that it was never my intention for you to read this book, find a glimmer of hope, and then put it aside. Instead, I want to challenge you to immediately take the next step in your wellbeing, and dare to try this one more treatment. To see if you are a candidate for my 21st Century Proprietary Pain Elimination Protocols, call our concierge clinic 24 hours a day, seven days a week at (888) 716-6028, email dryoo@lasermedinstitute.com or make an appointment online at www.lasermedinstitute.com.

Our 5-star quality of care and reputation for success has given prominent members of your community the confidence to come see us. We have treated Olympic Athletes, NFL Football and Major League Baseball players; highest-ranking military personnel and Special Forces units; Hollywood celebrities, musicians, entertainers, supermodels, and other high-profile individuals that were seeking fast relief, and found it. This has given our practice a higher profile, and caused us to only be able to accept a limited amount of cases.

I encourage you to take advantage of our accessibility and availability. Patients travel here from around the globe because our Lasermed Pain Institute is the only one in the world offering access to the world's most powerful Lifelite 60- and 250-watt Class IV lasers, along with my 21st Century Proprietary Pain Elimination Protocols.

Understandably, there are only a limited number of pain patients that can be seen, and there is often a two-week waiting list just to get in for an initial candidacy consultation.

It is critical that we do not exceed our capacity in order to preserve the quality of our care and service. We value the time that we spend with each patient so that we can do a thorough review of your unique situation to see if you are a candidate for our proprietary procedures, and so we can create a custom treatment plan designed to give you the fastest results possible if you do qualify.

Let There Be Hope

But there is still a place for you.

I encourage you to come take a tour of our concierge clinic in Southern California and see if you agree that this is the next step for you to take in your health care. As you will see in the following pages, we have an amazing track record with the cases we accept. We have successfully treated those suffering from fibromyalgia, carpal tunnel, shingles, failed surgeries, tendinitis, neuropathy, chronic pain, arthritis, and much, much more. We even have Home Therapy Programs for those unable to visit the institute for continuing care. If you would like to learn more about our concierge clinical services, or if you are a licensed health care professional* and would like to find out how to convert your practice into a "concierge clinic", then visit www.theconciergeclinic.com.

I understand that you may be exhausted and disheartened from all of your past failed attempts at finding relief. However, I have consistently found that 90.1% or more of the people that walk through my door can be helped. And almost 100% of those people are the last of the last; we are their last resort. I mention this because I want you to realize that these statistics are catered to your exact demographic.

If you have tried everything and nothing has worked, you are not alone. It has already been your experience that you are the exception to the rules; you do not benefit from the other treatments and modalities that you see others benefiting from. Perhaps things that have worked for you in the past have stopped working, or maybe you choose to believe that there is a better way out there.

Whatever your reasons are for stepping outside of the shadow of the pain you're living in, I want to assure you that I will be there to greet you, and to hopefully welcome you back to your active, pain free life.

*A Note to Physicians

I have been training doctors all around the world on my proprietary protocols in order to make the treatment available to more people suffering from chronic pain. If you are a medical doctor, chiropractor, physical therapist, or other licensed health care professional and the Class IV laser is under your scope of practice, you may register for one of my upcoming continuing education laser seminars, where you will get hands-on training with our Class IV lasers and earn re-licensing credits. (Check your state board requirements on attending 12 hours of re-licensing credits for laser physiotherapy sponsored by Logan College of Chiropractic Post Graduate Education Department.) Starting in 2013, most re-licensing credits will be cross-professional. Go to www.lasermedinstitute.com to register for our next laser seminar. You may email me (the dean & founder of the Lasermed Pain Institute post graduate education) at dryoo@lasermedinstitute.com.

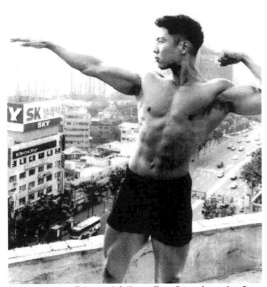

Here is my "Arnold Pose" a few days before the Mr. Seoul, Korea Bodybuilding Contest.

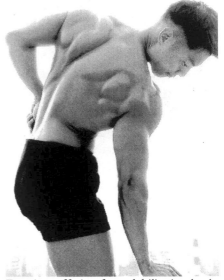

Despite suffering from debilitating back pain, I was able to overcome the disc problems and develop a strong and healthy back.

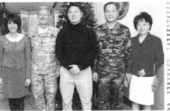

MILITARY GENERALS REVEAL THEIR TOP SECRET WEAPON FOR FIGHTING CHRONIC PAIN

Local Doctor Offers O.C. Veterans & Residents His Proprietary Pain Elimination Protocols Once Only Available To Top Military Officials, Special Forces, And Olympic Athletes.

One of the greatest honors during my time in Korea was receiving an Award of Appreciation from the top 4-star generals there. Here I am standing between General Sharp and General Lee at the "White House Christmas Party" in the capital city (Seoul) before receiving the award.

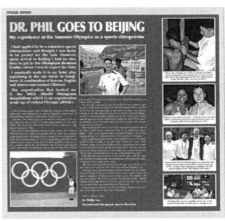

I treated athletes competing in the 2008 Olympic Games in Beijing, where I worked with retired legends like the World Olympians Association President Dick Fosbury, who invented the "Fosbury Flop" high jump technique and won the 1968 Gold medal in Mexico. Pictured next to him in the third image down on the right.

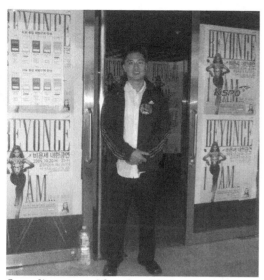

Standing outside the VIP entrance of the Beyoncé Tour before treating the back stage staff and performers.

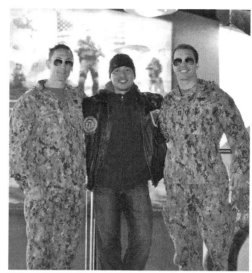

Here I am in my top gun jacket feeling safe and secure between two Navy Seals whom I sponsor by providing my laser therapy services.

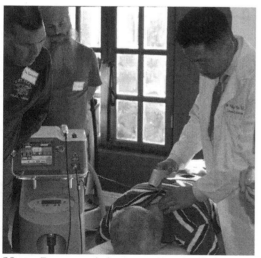

Here I am training a group of doctors on the use of the SRA infrared thermo scanner to detect pain, inflammation, and where to apply the world's most hi-powered Class IV laser to treat disc, nerve, joint, and soft tissue disorders.

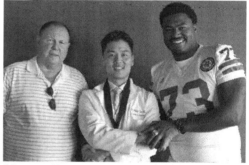

Here I am congratulating Bob Schellenberg (retired catcher for the Philadelphia Phillies), and DJ Jones (former NFL Baltimore Ravens Tackle) after successful clinical trial outcomes with the hi-powered laser. The laser helped Bob walk again, despite a bout of Chemotherapy, Parkinson's, and Diabetic Neuropathy. The laser decompression also helped DJ recover from a severe herniated disc and sciatica.

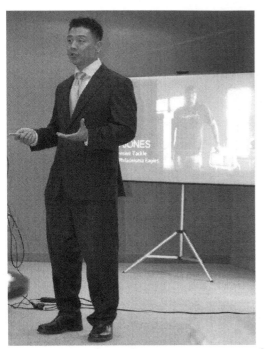

Here I am lecturing to a group of doctors about how DJ Jones (NFL player) was successfully treated with the hi-powered laser for his low back disc and sciatic pain.

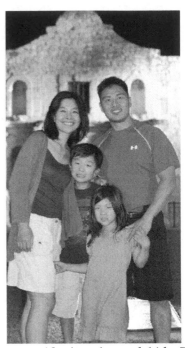

With my wife Angela, and kids David and Kathy at the Alamo after an International Church of Christ World Conference. I must like last stands since I am a die-hard Spartan.

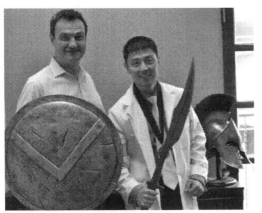

With Alan, fellow Michigan State Alumnus. I am your Spartan Pain Killer and will fight for you to the end. Aroo!

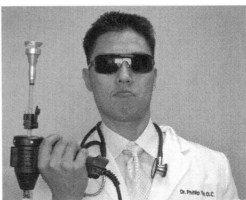

Dr. Phillip Yoo as "The Laser Pain Terminator."

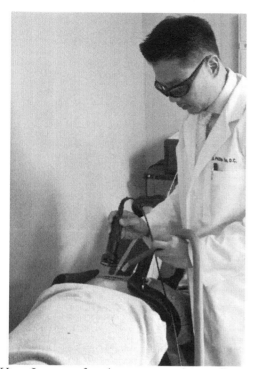

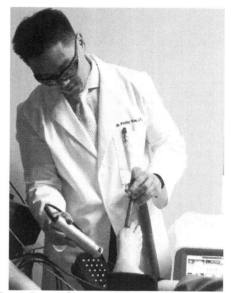

Here I perform my proprietary peripheral neuropathy relief protocol with the world's most powerful FDA cleared Class IV warm laser.

Here I am performing my proprietary disc & back pain laser decompression protocol with the world's most powerful class IV heated laser.

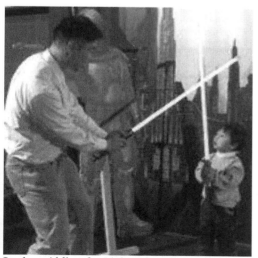

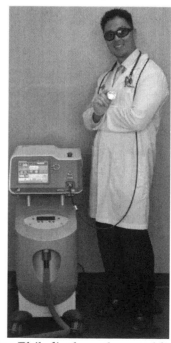

In the middle of a Light saber duel with my son David Luke when he was just 2 years old. "Use the Force, Luke!"

Dr. Phil displays the world's most powerful Class IV heated laser.

Part II
Conditions
&
Treatments

*"Is there no balm in Gilead? Is there no physician there? Why then is there no **healing** for the wound of my people?"*

-Jeremiah 8:22

Chapter 6

Medical Failures

Our Lasermed Pain Institute specializes in treating those who are suffering from chronic pain and have not responded to drugs, injections, surgery, or physical therapy; nor have they been helped by any other forms of alternative treatments such as acupuncture, chiropractic, herbal medicines, etc. Our typical patient has been to every specialist in town: the Dr. Rosens, the Dr. Bergs, the Dr. Steins, the Dr. Kims, the Dr. Lees; this neurologist, that neurologist; this pain management specialist, that pain management specialist – but are still suffering from ridiculous pain!

Like most people who suffer from chronic pain, your first stop is likely to by your primary care doctor, who will usually prescribe you some sort of painkiller that merely blocks the pain signals that go to your brain, at best. When that doesn't work, the physician will refer you to a pain management specialist, who will either prescribe more powerful pain-killing pills, or prolotherapy, corticosteroid, or epidural injections – hit-or-miss invasive procedures that carry some risk with them. When that fails, you are usually referred to a neurologist or orthopedic surgeon, who may prescribe a nerve block, morphine pump, or even high-risk surgical procedure.

The problem with these procedures is that they all carry significant risk to your health and well-being. The prescription pain medications usually have to be taken long term, and have undesirable side effects on your kidneys, liver, digestion, and nervous systems. They can even be fatal; more people have died taking prescription medications than in car accidents! Furthermore, injections have been shown to be a high-risk procedure, as they may result in permanent nerve damage if the needle punctures the wrong structure, and certain patients may have adverse side effects to the drugs being injected.

Lastly, the failure rate for back surgeries is much higher than one can imagine, and may result in permanent disability if the surgeon cuts the wrong structure. In fact, some of you may have even experienced a failed surgery, which has led to repeated surgical procedures, or having the surgical hardware removed. This is something we seen often in our clinic, and we're happy to report that we have been able to use the laser to successfully treat and help manage many of these failed cases like yours.

Case Studies

"After six sessions, I would say I'm completely cured!"

Painful Knees with Numbness and Swelling
Due to Past Sports Injury

"I'm 76 years old and from Fountain Valley, CA. I was a sportsman who has had several injuries, one of which was a bad knee accident resulting in a knee replacement. The problem was that I have had bad circulation, mainly in my right foot, which gave me numbness at nighttime, a lot of pain, inability to sleep on the right side at night, and swollen feet. All the doctors did was prescribe me pain pills, but obviously it was just a Band-Aid approach to the problem. I saw Dr. Yoo's ad in the paper on laser technology and I made an appointment to come in for a consultation and to start some treatments. After the first couple treatments, the pain in my hips went away, my numbness went away, the circulation in my feet were much improved, and after six sessions, I would say I'm completely cured. I would recommend this technology and treatment to anybody who has this type of pain.

Bill Melnik, Fountain Valley, CA

(See Bill's amazing story by typing in "Bill can walk again laser" into the YouTube.com search bar.)

"Today I'm actually pain-free. It's like a miracle!"

<u>Doctor's Torn Meniscus Relief After Trying: Prolotherapy,
Chiropractic, Electric Therapy, and Acupuncture</u>

"I've been a Beverly Hills chiropractor for 23 years. I injured my knee about two months ago in a pretty bad accident that resulted in a torn meniscus and was in severe pain. I had many different treatments ranging from prolotherapy, magnetic therapy, electric therapy, chiropractic, and acupuncture, but nothing really got rid of the pain. I finally heard about Dr. Yoo and the laser therapy online and decided to try it out. I've had three treatments on my knee, and this weekend was the first weekend I was actually able to go exercise. Today I'm actually pain-free. It's like a miracle because I actually was considering surgery. I'm extremely pleased with the results, and I'm actually going to buy one of these lasers for myself.

Dr. Harhari Khalsa, Beverly Hills, CA

(See the doctor's amazing story by typing "Dr. Harhari, avoids meniscus surgery laser" into the YouTube.com search bar.)

"The swelling has gone down dramatically, the cramping has relieved, and I'm able to function a lot better than I was before."

<u>Inflammation, Swelling, Pain, & Cramping in Legs
Due to Long Periods of Standing</u>

"I am an educator so I tend to be on my feet often. I have severe inflammation in my legs to the point where I had Dopplers done to see if there were any signs of blood clotting. I've been prescribed drugs, but nothing seemed to give me any relief. A friend of mine referred me to Dr. Yoo's clinic, and upon the first treatment I saw a real difference in the swelling of my legs. On my second treatment, I was able to wear shoes that I haven't been able to fit in for the last two years. Due to the cramping, pain, and swelling in my legs the past couple of years I had to buy shoes in all different sizes in order to feel comfortable. After the treatments these past couple of weeks, I feel as though the swelling has gone down dramatically, the cramping has relieved, and I'm able to function a lot better than I was before. I'm very appreciative for these treatments and I plan on continuing and getting to a full recovery.

Louise Sobieski, Mission Viejo, CA

(See her raving review by typing "Louise's laser" into the YouTube.com search bar.)

"I can see a change!"

Numbness in the Metatarsals, Bone Spur, & Pain in Primary Fascia After Seeing Podiatrist

"I saw Dr. Yoo's ad in the newspaper, and another friend had also told me that she came to see him. I have had this numbness in my feet, and I was really concerned about it. I had been to a podiatrist who just trimmed my nails; I told him I had this pain in my primary fascia, which he addressed with a cortisone shot about two years ago. The shot stopped the pain, but I still had numbness in my metatarsals. It's feeling better now after my laser treatments. I also have a bone spur that Dr. Yoo had been working on using the Graston technique. I really think it's helping me because I can see a change in the way it looks. Between that and the laser, I'm hoping this bone spur goes away. I was thinking I would need an operation on my feet due to the spur, so I'm hoping this will help me avoid it."

Eleanor Bryant, Costa Mesa, CA

(See her amazing story by typing "Eleanor avoids food operation laser" into the YouTube.com search bar.)

Chapter 7

Chronic Back Pain

(See also Arthritis, Bugling Disc, Degenerative Disc Disease, Herniated Disc, Sciatica)

Back pain can be a persistent thorn in your side, affecting every motion throughout your day. This may go from a dull, throbbing ache to a sudden sharp pain that takes your breath away. For some, this experience may onset suddenly and last for just a few miserable days, while others have the misfortune of suffering for an extended period of time. This could stretch into months, and even years.

If you find yourself suffering for longer than three months, then you are struggling with chronic back pain.

If this describes you, you have certainly taken measures to stem the pain. You may have had limited success with over-the-counter pain relievers, but you probably also recognize that this simply offers a small window of relief, and that the pain not only returns, but continues to worsen. You may have instinctively started restricting your movement or be spending prolonged periods of time in bed. The irony, though, is that this only agitates the situation and increases the pain.

Identifying the Onset and Symptoms

You'll usually first feel back pain just after you lift a heavy object, move suddenly, sit in one position for a long time, or have an injury or accident. Acute low back pain is most often caused by a sudden injury to the muscles, ligaments, bones, and nerves in the spine.

Symptoms include:

- Tingling and prickling or burning sensations.
- Sharp shooting pains.

- Dull persistent aching.
- Throbbing and burning.
- Shaking and limb weakness.
- Intense leg pain.
- Inability to bend or lift.
- Pain or discomfort sitting for extended periods of time.

What To Do

At this point, you have probably already found some treatments that offer some temporary relief and reduce inflammation, like applying heat or ice packs and taking over-the-counter pain relievers. Although they may help to manage your daily suffering by giving you a few hours of relief, they will not go to the root of the cause and keep the pain from coming back. It's the age-old problem of treating the symptoms of the problem, but not the problem itself. For instance, if a skunk keeps squeezing through a hole in your fence and spraying your dog, you can choose to (A) invest in expensive air fresheners, or (B) patch the hole and keep the skunk from coming back.

At the Lasermed Pain Institute, we use techniques to go to the source of the problem, and heal the root cause, instead of just temporarily treating the symptoms (the band aid approach). Our Proprietary Lifelite Laser Protocols treat the root cause of your disease, which immediately relieves the symptoms of your pain, numbness, and inflammation.

There are several things you can do at home in order to complement our therapies. These things include:

- **Rest** - If your back hurts too much, take a break; but try not to let too much time pass before you get moving again. Instead, return to your activities slowly, and avoid things that make your pain worse. Studies show that bed rest doesn't relieve back pain better than staying active. And bed rest of more than a couple of days can make your back pain worse and lead to other problems, such as stiff joints and muscle weakness.
- **Use a heating pad or ice pack** - Heat can reduce pain and stiffness. Ice can help reduce pain and swelling, and should be used for at least the first 48 hours of the onset of pain. You

might want to switch back and forth between heat and cold until you find what helps you the most. (When in doubt use ice on the painful or injured area for 20 minutes on and off until the pain subsides.)

- **Exercise** - Ask your doctor or a physical therapist about what kinds of exercises you can do to stretch and strengthen the muscles in your back, shoulders, and stomach. These muscles help support your spine. Strong muscles can help improve your posture, keep your body in better balance, decrease your chance of injury, and reduce pain.

- **Practice good posture** - Poor posture puts stress on your back. Be sure to stand or sit tall, with your shoulders and your stomach pulled in to support your back. Don't slump or slouch.

- **Learn ways to reduce stress** - Stress can make your pain feel worse. You might try deep breathing and relaxation exercises or meditation. You may also consider seeing a counselor because cognitive-behavioral therapy can show you how to change certain thoughts and behaviors to control your pain.

- **Eat a nutritious diet** - Getting plenty of calcium and vitamin D may help prevent osteoporosis, which can lead to compression fractures and back pain.

- **Don't smoke** - Smoking decreases blood flow and slows healing.

- **Take extra care when lifting** - When you must lift, bend your knees and keep your back straight. Avoid twisting. Keep the load close to your body.

- **Use a pain diary** - Write down how your moods, thoughts, sleep patterns, activities, and medicines affect your pain. Having a record of your pain can help us find the best ways to treat it.

- **Avoid prolonged bed rest -** This just makes it worse.

- **Find out if you are a candidate for laser decompression** - My proprietary back pain elimination protocols have saved many patients from pain and surgery. Go to www.ocspinedisc.com, or call (888) 716-6028 to find out if you are a candidate.

Case Studies

"Five years of pain have gone away, and I am now able to sleep through the night."

<u>Back Pain Due to College Football After Trying Acupuncture, Physical Therapy, and Muscular Therapy</u>

"I just started getting treatments by Dr. Yoo for the past month. I played football for USC for about five years. During my time in college football, I developed a pretty severe back problem. None of the treatments were effective at the school. I saw a bunch of specialists, but they had no conclusive diagnosis. Since graduating, I've sought out acupuncture therapy, muscular therapy, physical therapy, and pretty much anything you could do. Unfortunately, nothing would help in any way. I was at the end of my rope and sprung on the article about Dr. Yoo. This was the last treatment I was going to try before back surgery, and since I've started with Dr. Yoo, my back has improved dramatically. Five years of pain have gone away, and I am now able to sleep through the night, which is something I wasn't able to do before. I can work out a lot more actively than I was able to before, and I feel much better. I always wanted to serve my country and become a Navy Seal. Now that my back problem is under control, going to BUDS training just might become a reality.

Spencer Vigoren, USC Football Alumni, Laguna Beach, CA

(You can see Spencer's raving review by typing "USC low back pain laser" into the YouTube.com search bar.)

"My back feels much, much better, and I can go back to work again!"

<u>Unable to Work Because of Chronic Back Pain</u>

"I have been suffering for 15 or more years with back problems. I tried everything: acupuncture, chiropractors, and nothing helped. One day I was reading the newspaper and saw Dr. Yoo's ad. So I came in to make an appointment. After the first treatment, I felt 50% better than I had before, and the second treatment I felt completely better. At

this point, from a level of one to 10, my pain is down to three or four, and I'm feeling like I can go back to work. I'm currently not working because of my problems, but now I feel much, much, much better with this treatment.

Alberto Aguilar, Anaheim, CA

(You can see Alberto's review by typing "Alberto's Back Pain Cure" into the YouTube.com search bar.)

"I'm a believer, let me tell you!"
Chronic Back Pain, Even After Trying Epidurals and More

"I came in for lower back pain, which was at about an eight. I had tried epidurals and all kinds of other things. My range of motion was such that I could barely bend at the waist. After one treatment [with decompression and the laser], when I left, I could almost touch my toes. It makes me cry to think about it! I can stand and walk for half an hour with no pain. I'm a believer, let me tell you!"

Susan Gabriel, Irvine, CA

(You can see Susan's raving review by typing "Susan's Back Pain Cure" into the YouTube.com search bar.)

Chapter 8

Bulging Discs

When patients come to my office with bulging discs, I can often tell before I even ask for their symptoms. Their contorted bodies tell all. They bend this way and that, seeking relief from the painful deformity along their spine.

Although it is one of the more painful and acute conditions that plague my patients, it is also one of the easiest to treat and correct. I have consistently been able to relieve the symptoms and help eliminate the root cause of the problem. When athletes come to my office for treatment, this is most often the reason. (I talked earlier about the NFL player, DJ Jones, that came to my office for multiple reasons, one of which was a bulging disc.) But you don't have to be an athlete to be affected by this painful problem, as you well know.

(To see the most powerful Class IV hi-powered laser in action as it is used to treat the disc of our 6'5", 310-pound Pro Football Player, type "Pro Football Player, decompression laser therapy" into the YouTube.com search bar.)

What It Is

A bulging disc is not the same as a herniated disc, although some of the symptoms and characteristics are the same. Where a herniated disc is a rupture in the outer layer of the disc, causing the gel-like inside of the disc to bulge out of its protective casing, a bulging disc actually bulges out from between the vertebrae where it rests. It can press on the spinal cord and nerves, causing mild to intense pain.

Identifying Onset and Symptoms

The pain that comes from a bulging disc is similar to the pain of a herniated disc, in that it is more severe when you are in motion, and is reduced when you are still. Even little, daily motions like coughing, sneezing, bending, and driving can intensify the pain. The reason for this is that as you move, you are putting more pressure on the nerve.

The pain will not always manifest itself in the area of the bulging disc. The nerves that are being affected can spread pain through larger areas of the body, and you may mistakenly believe that the problem is in those other areas. For instance, if the disc is putting pressure on the nerves associated with the legs, you may have shooting pain through the legs or your feet may go numb. It would only be natural for you to fear there is something wrong with your limbs, since that's where the symptoms are occurring.

Symptoms may include:

- Mild or intense back pain.
- Shooting pains spreading through one or both legs.
- Sharp pain when twisting your upper body to the left or right.
- Trouble controlling your limbs.
- Loss of balance.
- Numbness and tingling in your feet and/or legs.
- Pain when you move or lift your arms or legs.
- Sciatic symptoms.

What To Do

You have probably already sought some kind of relief, with or without temporary success. However, the only lasting relief comes from identifying and fixing the problem. You can take pain relievers all day long, but you can be sure that this is just putting a Band-Aid over the problem.

You should immediately schedule an appointment by emailing us at info@ocspinedisc.com, calling our concierge clinic at (888) 716-6028, or making an appointment online at www.ocspinedisc.com to find out if you are a candidate for our Laser Decompression treatment to begin healing the disc. This is the best method for both relieving the symptoms, and eliminating the problems. The decompression therapy will gently pull the vertebrae apart, eventually restoring the normal pump mechanism of the disc. This will restore water in the dehydrated disc, and help cause the disc to go back in between the vertebrae and immediately take the pressure off the nerves. Coupling this with the hi-powered Laser Therapy brings the healing photonic energy to the area, which heals and strengthens the damaged disc, nerve and vertebrae.

Case Study

"I am back to playing volleyball and my pain level is at a low."

<u>College Volleyball Player with a Protruding L4 and L5</u>

"I came in with a protruding L4 and L5 lumbar. Basically, it is the worst pain I have ever experienced. I play volleyball for my college, and this pain began in April of last year. I really did not think much of it. So around that June, I started to seek help from different doctors and chiropractors. The doctors told me to do stretches and pain relieving exercises, but nothing was helping me; my pain was still there. I even signed up for physical therapy and it still was not helping me. So, one day my girlfriend heard about Dr. Yoo on the radio, so I came in with a pain level of six to eight. And after having the laser and decompression treatments, I am back to playing volleyball and my pain level now is at a low two. This treatment has done so much more for me than physical therapy. Thank you to my girlfriend for listening to the radio. And thank you to Dr. Yoo for helping me get back to the sport I love to play.

Harley Frost, San Juan Capistrano, CA

(You can see Harley's video testimonial by typing "Harland improves back pain" into the YouTube.com search bar.)

62

Chapter 9

Herniated Discs

Herniated discs are painful, and may require you to put an abrupt halt to your life until it can be resolved. Those who suffer may be struggling with the fear of surgery, as they are unsuccessful in their search for relief. Pain killers only mask the pain and do nothing to correct the structural problem with the body.

If left untreated, it can lead to additional trauma to the spine and body, loss of work and wages, and a huge reduction in the quality of your life.

What It Is

If you have a herniated disc, you have a tear in the outer, fibrous ring of your disc. This tear allows the gel-like pulposa to leak from the center and push against the disc's outer wall. If it ruptures, a chemical is released that causes the nerves to swell. If left untreated, it can lead to other physical issues like pinched nerves, bulging discs, and sciatica.

A herniated disc can be caused by a variety of things, from regular wear and tear on the body, to a traumatic physical injury. A hernia can be found anywhere along the spine, although it is most often found in the lower back area, or the lumbar region. If it is located in the cervical or neck area, it can lead to dizziness, severe tension headaches, and pain in the shoulders, arms, and neck.

Identifying Onset and Symptoms:

Not all herniated discs are painful. In fact, they are most often detected only after they have caused other physical issues, like pinched nerves and sciatica, which have a wide spectrum of physical manifestations. (You can view those symptoms in their relevant chapters.) X-rays and MRIs can be used to detect herniated discs, but these are not always reliable, since the tear in the disc may not be big enough to detect.

What To Do

You should immediately schedule an appointment by calling our concierge clinic at (888) 716-6028, emailing us at info@ocspinedisc.com, or making an appointment online at www.ocspinedisc.com, to find out if you are a candidate for our Laser Decompression treatment, which will immediately begin healing the disc. Be sure to bring any X-rays, CT scans, or MRIs to your consultation so that we can get a thorough picture of your unique situation.

Our Laser Decompression treatment alleviates the pressure on the affected site, and gently opens the correlating vertebrae. This pumps in nourishing blood and spinal fluid into the area, and makes the damaged disc more accessible to the photonic energy coming from the laser, which is equivalent to the life-giving rays of the sun.

This treatment causes your body's natural healing mechanisms to magnify and seal up the injured disc. The tissue fibers knit together, sealing off the tear, and restoring the disc to full health. Any peripheral health issues that may have cropped up as a result of the herniated disc are also simultaneously treated.

Case Study

"To have the laser done right after decompression was heaven."

Herniated Discs and a Ripped Shoulder After Falling

"I was fine throughout my life until I had a terrible fall that completely threw me off. I had herniated discs and a shoulder that ripped; I had to have surgery. At first my spine did not bother me, but as time passed it started to give me this excruciating pain. All the doctors I saw only prescribed pain medications. It was like they were taking my wounds and wrapping them in bandages. One day I was reading the LA Times and saw Dr. Phillip Yoo's ad on decompression and laser

treatment and his testimonial on what was going on with his own body and how these treatments helped him. Everything that Dr. Yoo spoke about that was happening with him was the exact thing that I was going through. After my first session, I came off the decompression table feeling so amazing, a feeling I have not felt in so long. To have the laser done right after decompression was heaven. My second session was even more amazing. The third session, I had two decompressions, one on my neck and one on my back. When I got off the decompression and laser treatment for my back, I felt even more ecstatic. Let me be the first to say this to all of you out there who may be suffering with the same pain: come and see Dr. Phillip Yoo. His treatments work! Thank you Dr. Yoo for helping me get rid of all the pain that has been my companion for so many years."

Nettie Gonzales, Los Angeles, CA

Chapter 10

Degenerative Disc Disease

Disc degeneration will happen to all of us over time without proper treatment. Your discs are constantly being used over the course of your life, and degeneration is just part of the aging process. However, not everyone will, or has to, develop symptoms that will interfere with their daily lives. I have seen patients get out of pain their condition dramatically improve.

What It Is

Degenerative disc disease is the result of the body's natural aging process. When we are born, our spinal discs are made up of about 80% water. This is what gives the disc the spongy quality that allows it to absorb the shock of our daily activities. Over time, however, the amount of water in the disc is reduced, and it becomes less spongy. This, in turn, means that it does not absorb as much shock, and that pressure is rerouted to other areas of the body.

Through the aging process, the proteins in the disc space also begin to change, often leading to tears in the outer protection of the disc called the annulus fibrosus. Most of us will have some level of disc degeneration by the time we reach 60, without pain.

In severe case, the degeneration is accompanied by disabling pain.

Identifying Onset and Symptoms

An MRI or X-ray will give you a clear picture of how much your discs have degenerated. Most people will not pursue this information unless they are part of the minority that is suffering. Onset for the typical active person will be during the mid-30s or 40s. Associated pain will usually be fleeting and low grade.

Symptoms include:

- The presence of low back pain, agitated when sitting, bending, lifting, and twisting.
- A decrease of pain when walking and even running.
- Lying down helps to eliminate the pain, since this relieves stress on the disc space.

Severe back pain related to degenerative disc disease will generally last from a few days to a few months before the patient's pain subsides to the baseline level of chronic discomfort. The pain can be disabling and keep you from performing your regular, daily activities.

What To Do

You should immediately schedule an appointment by calling our concierge clinic at (888) 716-6028 emailing us at info@ocspinedisc.com, or making an appointment online at www.ocspinedisc.com, to find out if you are a candidate for our Laser Decompression treatment, and to begin healing your degenerated disc disease.

The Class IV hi-powered laser may help to relieve your painful symptoms and aid your body in healing the affected area and return you to your normal life. The laser penetrates the area, delivering a powerful blast of safe, photonic energy. This nurtures the area, the same way the sun does. In fact, it's utilizing the same natural process the sun uses to give your body vitamin D3. It induces greater circulation and cell reproduction, which helps to knit the tears and splits in the degenerated disc so that they heal.

After it is determined you are a candidate for the Laser Decompression procedure and you are out of acute pain, we graduate you to a spinal rehabilitation program that includes regular exercise for faster healing and better disc health. This might seem counterintuitive, since you may fear that the added activity will cause faster degeneration. In fact, the disc and the spinal area were made to constantly move in order to keep the spinal joints lubricated and discs hydrated with water. Sitting stagnant for too long can cause greater low back pain as spinal joints get stiff and discs dehydrate. This inactivity also causes your body to gain weight, which increases the work load of each disc and joint.

A regular routine of back exercises can prevent low back pain and/or reduce the severity and duration of any "flare-ups." Controlled, gradual, progressive back pain exercises can help the back retain its strength and flexibility.

In our clinic, we use spinal decompression combined with hi-powered lasers to help the healing process along and to give your back the additional movement it needs. This therapy uses a rhythmic extending action to help open up your vertebrae and bring life-giving blood, water, and spinal fluid into the spinal joints and discs. (The absorption of water into the disc with this pumping mechanism is called "imbibition".) This helps to pump the disc up with fluids to counter the effects of the degenerated vertebrae collapsing on each other and will help to nourish the area for faster relief. In opening up the vertebrae in this way, we are also able to ensure that the laser therapy is able to penetrate as deeply as possible, bringing the photonic energy deep into the problem areas for faster results.

Furthermore, after your pain is eliminated, we graduate our disc patients to the rehabilitative phase, where we strengthen the core muscles in the stomach and back, and increase your functional spinal range of motion, by using a special device called an ATM (Active Therapeutic Motion) to minimize the shearing forces that damage the disc tissue. The ATM machine was originally developed to improve functional range of motion to professional golfers to help them drive the ball further. Now, its use has expanded into other sports and is often used in rehabilitating those with dysfunctional movement patterns, as found in disc pain patients.

(To see how the ATM restores a pain-free range of motion in a Professional athlete, type "Pro Volleyball amazing results ATM" into the YouTube.com search bar.)

Case Studies

"I have been feeling a lot better."

Degenerative Disc Disease on Cervical Spine

"I am an Internist Pulmonologist by Craning practicing for the last 45 years. I also teach at USC and White Memorial, and I am currently the director of both hospitals. I decided to see Dr. Yoo because of my chronic, severe neck pain and left shoulder pain. He diagnosed me with degenerative disease on my cervical spine and left shoulder. He decided that laser treatment and decompression would be beneficial to my chronic pain. Since I came a month ago, I have been feeling a lot better in this process. So I would like to say I'm doing better with this treatment.

Reynaldo Landero, M.D., Los Angeles, CA

(You can see the good doctor's testimonial by typing "Dr. Reynaldo neck laser treatment"" into YouTube.com's search bar.)

"I did my first laser treatment and there was no pain at all!"

Degenerated Disc Pain - Lumbar

"My name is Gary Conrad from Newport Beach, CA. I had my first laser treatment a few days ago for my lower back pain. I was extremely skeptical if the treatment would work. I have tried everything you can think of; epidurals, acupuncture, and chiropractors but nothing ever really worked. I did my first laser treatment, and afterwards there was no pain whatsoever. In fact, it actually felt great. When I got off the table the pain was gone, I kept waiting for the pain to return and it has not returned. A lot of people would say that I shuffle when I walk, but ever since the treatment I have not been shuffling."

Gary Conrad, Newport, CA

(You can see Gary's transformation by typing "Gary's laser back pain" into the YouTube.com search bar.)

Chapter 11

Failed Back Surgery Treatment

Most of my patients are those who have tried everything to find relief and come up empty handed. Often, I am the last hope before someone resorts to surgery, which is often considered the most extreme and invasive way you can possibly seek a solution. Unfortunately, there are even those who have already tried surgery, and are still left to suffer.

Even though I have suffered from multiple debilitating conditions in my lifetime, I have been able to avoid surgery. My desire to do so was one of the things that finally lead me to discover the current laser therapy I use in my practice. At the time, I was motivated by a determination to avoid such an invasive procedure if at all possible.

I can only imagine the discouragement and hopelessness that must come after a failed surgery – that which was supposed to be the last resort. I am so grateful to have found a way to both help people avoid surgery, and to give those who have already gone through surgery another reason to hope.

What It Is

Following surgeries, other disorders can develop into a "musical chairs" scenario of disorders involving the affected area. We call this "Pain Roulette," as patients struggle to discover what the next most effective "magic bullet" will be to solve their pain issues.

Symptoms

Following surgery, you may find that there are other pains developing that were not there before; or that the pain you were seeking to get rid of has returned. Some patients also experience an increasing dependence on, and eventually even an addiction to, painkilling drugs as they try to cope with the disorder by making their body unaware of the real problem.

Symptoms may include:

- Numbness and/or loss of sensitivity.
- Tingling and a prickling or burning sensation.
- Sharp pains and cramps.
- Difficulty sitting or standing for long periods of time.
- Loss of balance or coordination.
- Bell's Palsy on one side of the face.

What To Do

If you think you have a failed surgery response, you should immediately schedule an appointment by calling our concierge clinic at (888) 716-6028, or emailing us at info@ocspinedisc.com.

I may be able to help you, but it's important for you to contact us as soon as possible. We treat many kinds of recurring and re-developing pains, and can detect if you may need deep medical attention, while providing relief for immediate pain. We use the Lifelite Laser Neuropathy Elimination Protocols to relieve neuropathic pain, and to bombard the affected areas with healing photonic energy. This energy penetrates deep into your tissues and stimulates the body's natural healing mechanisms to get to work. The process is very much like one the sun uses to produce Vitamin D3 in your body.

This process is non-invasive and may be able to give you immediate relief.

Case Studies

"A good night's sleep at last."

<u>Degenerative Disc. Peripheral Neuropathy, & Bladder Dysfunction with Failed Back Surgery</u>

"I have been through a series of back operations, beginning with a laminectomy, and then eventually the doctors decided to put in metal parts. It's been extremely painful to go through the process, and over a

period of time, it has not solved the problem. Right now, I rely upon pills to control the pain, but I was tempted to find a better solution and I responded to the advertisements for these laser treatments. After three treatments, there has certainly been an improvement for the amount of pain during the day. The amount of times I have had to urinate at night has dramatically decreased from four to six times a night to only two. I consider the treatments to have been greatly helpful for me getting a good night's sleep."

Richard Mills, Claremont, CA

(You see Richard's transformation by typing "Richard's failed back surgery laser" into the YouTube.com search bar.)

"I am able to get out of bed feeling much better & my physical activity has been increasing!"

<u>Low Back Pain/ Spinal Stenosis / Fused Neck</u>

I was guided here very providentially to receive some decompression and laser treatment with Dr. Phillip Yoo. I have suffered with low back pain, stenosis & vertebral problems for many years because of a birth congenital condition when I was born. I have been to many orthopedic doctors and orthopedic surgeons. I had to have a fusion surgery on my neck where three vertebrates had to be fused because I had problems there. I was told by three surgeons that I will need to have a lumbar surgery for the condition that I have with my lower back. I have been suffering from so much pain issues, as well as tingling and numbness. In the past, I tried so many different pain medications to relive the excruciating pain I was feeling. I was fortunate to come and see Dr. Phillip Yoo and his non-invasive laser treatment center. I received decompression on the KDT decompression machine, and more importantly I have had laser treatment to my back with the LRX 60-watt laser in the affected areas. After just two weeks of treatment, much pain has been alleviated. I am able to get out of bed feeling much better. My physical activity has been increasing, especially cycling. I am hoping that with more of these treatments, it will eliminate my long-standing chronic back pain. I am so happy to be here with such a professional doctor who is helping a lot of individuals such as myself.

Thank you so much Dr. Phillip Yoo. I feel so fortunate to be a candidate for this treatment."

Terrence Tribbey, Fountain Valley, CA

(See Terry's raving review by typing "Terry's terrific laser disc" into the YouTube.com search bar.)

"I am able to walk with the walker and my hip doesn't hurt as badly."

<u>Hip And Back Pain After</u>
<u>Diabetic Leg Amputation. Trying Pills,</u>
<u>Acupuncture, And Injections</u>

"I had a leg amputation about two years ago. I have not been able to walk with my prosthesis because it hurts too badly when I put weight on it. I have tried everything from injections, pain management, acupuncture, and whatever I could get ahold of. I saw the ad about the laser clinic and I thought this would be my last chance of getting any help. I've done about five treatments and now I am able to walk with the walker and my hip does not hurt as badly. Thank You Dr. Phil."

Lucille Robinson, Huntington Beach, CA

(See Lucy's amazing transformation by typing "Lucille's laser now she can sleep" into the YouTube.com search bar.)

"I have zero pain!"

<u>Bone-On-Bone Degenerative Knee Arthritis</u>

"Hello ladies and gentlemen. This is Alan Adler speaking to you from the Lasermed Institute in Costa Mesa, C.A. What I'm about to tell you is something that's very unbelievable. First of all, I have had knee trouble for probably the last ten years of my life. The cartilage in my knees has basically disintegrated. My knees are now bone on bone. As the years have gone on, it has been getting worse and worse. I went through the normal procedure of talking to orthopedic surgeons and taking medication for the pain. But the bottom line was that it didn't

help. I was looking for something new and something different. We are in the Twenty-First century, and I believe that there is a lot in the world of new technology that is just beginning to touch the surface in the medical field. I read an article in the Los Angeles Times about three months ago about the Lasermed Institute. I came in for an interview with Dr. Phillip Yoo, and we sat down for about forty five minutes. He examined me and it sounded like there was potential, so I said, "Let's try it."

At the end of the laser treatment, I got off the table — and you're not going to believe it but I hope you do because I'm telling you the truth — I had zero pain. Zero pain! Through the treatments each time, the pain becomes less and less throughout my entire body. I had pain in my shoulders, lower back, knees, calves, and also in my ankles. I now have almost zero pain in both knees, and before I was running around an eight or nine out of ten in pain consistently. I'm looking forward to a surprise for my fiancée by inviting her out for dinner at a dance hall. I'd love to show her that I can dance again, which has been my biggest ambition all along. I'm so excited about it. If you doubt that these things are possible, come in for your own consultation and examination, listen to what this man has to say, look at his program, look at the instruments he uses. Yes it's Buck Rogers, it's Twenty-First century, it's Dr. Spock; but truthfully it works!"

Alan Adler, Dana Point, CA (Former U.S. Navy Attack Pilot)

"After the first treatment, I noticed a huge difference."

<u>Osteoarthritis Of The Knees</u>

"I've been having trouble with my knees, and I couldn't get down on the floor with my grandkids to play. I've tried to teach them to jump rope, and I couldn't jump. When I went up and down the stairs it was difficult, so I came in to Dr. Yoo. After the first treatment, I noticed a huge difference. I could get down on the floor with the grandkids; I could actually sit there and play a game with them. And now after a few treatments I can go up and down the stairs without having to hold onto the railing to pull myself up, or to help myself get down. I can actually put my leg down and raise my body just with the strength in my knee without having to use my arm, which I haven't been able to do for a long time. I'm thrilled."

Sherry Kettley, Newport Beach, CA

"I'm pretty amazed with the laser and how it's helped me."

Torn Menisuc And Arthritis
From A Ski Accident

"Hi, I'm from Whittier, C.A. I met Dr. Yoo because my husband was coming to see him. While we were there, I said, "Hey, take a look at my knee." I suffered an alpine injury two years ago, and that resulted in what they call the unhappy triad. So ACL/MCL, meniscus, broken tibia head, and patella. The whole thing was quite traumatic for a while. I underwent surgery, ACL repair, and the MCL repaired on its own. I have just had really bad atrophy of the quad. I'm not in a good condition to take stairs, and my mobility was pretty limited. I did the laser treatments with Dr. Yoo, and it's a little addicting how good the hot treatment feels on the knee. I have much less pain overall. It has been fantastic for me to physically touch the scar site. The knee and my flexibility is painless. I still have some patella pain way below, but compared to when I started it's pretty amazing how it feels to physically touch that area. After six treatments, I'm pretty amazed with the laser and how it's helped me."

Terrilynn Salisbury, Whittier, CA

"I walked out of the clinic with no pain."

Failed Total Knee Replacement Surgeries

"I came in to see Dr. Yoo because I had several arthroscopic knee surgeries, and then each knee had to have a knee replacement. One of them failed, so they had to go back in and fix that. I've been to physical therapy, have tried pain medications, and have been through a couple of different knee surgeries. Finally, after the very first laser treatment I walked out of the clinic with no pain and I have been great since!"

Joyce French, Fullerton, CA

Chapter 12

Arthritis

Arthritis is one of the most rampant disabling diseases, with at least 10% of the world's population currently suffering. Many of those affected restrict their daily activities, with 750,000 Americans being unable to attend work, school, or perform daily functional tasks.

This means the quality of life is being consistently subjected to the dominance of the disease. There are violins gathering dust in the corner, grandchildren that are not being held, and vacations that will never be taken. This is not a lethal disease in terms of being the cause of physical death, but the amount of life being drained from the day-to-day existence coated in pain is not a great way to live, either.

Inflammation is one of the major symptoms of the disease, so this is often the target of treatment. While there are various popular methods used with a wide range of results, if you're reading this book you probably have not been satisfied with the previous treatment options you've been given. It may be that there are things that have worked well for you in the in the past, such as Prednisone, corticosteroid shots, TNF drugs, etc., but now you find that you are no longer responding to these treatments, and you are discouraged to find your life bound in debilitating pain once again.

Different Types of Arthritis

There are different types of arthritis, but each form of the disease has a similar effect on the lives of those that suffer. The pain and stiffness leads to the restriction of movement and the ability to do the things that once brought joy and signified vitality.

- **Rheumatoid Arthritis**

The onset period for Rheumatoid Arthritis is usually before the age of 45. This disease deforms the bones and joints through inflammation caused by substances found in the blood.

- **Osteoarthritis**

The onset period of Osteoarthritis is usually after the age of 45, and is a result of age. Forty-five years of activity can put a lot of "wear and tear" on the human body, with the joints and tendons taking the brunt of the baggage. This results in severe inflammation.

- **Spinal Osteoarthritis**

Osteoarthritis can sometimes manifest itself as another form of the disease called spinal osteoarthritis. This is when there is a breakdown of the cartilage of the joints and discs in the lower back and neck. This is often accompanied by painful bone spurs, called osteophytes, which put pressure on the nerves. Another form of osteoarthritis is degenerative disc disease, which brings on another set of problems and necessary physical restrictions.

Identifying Onset and Symptoms

Those who are starting to develop arthritis may first notice a measure of stiffness when they walk, and in the movement of the hands and feet. You may also experience dull aches and pains throughout the body without being able to identify exactly where they are coming from. You may notice inflamed joints, marked by pain and redness or swelling. These symptoms may be accompanied by mild physical fatigue, a weak grip in the hands, and other muscle weakness that may make you feel unbalanced when you're walking or standing.

Symptoms include:

- Thick feeling in the fingers and the inability to make a fist.
- Stiffness in the joints: legs, feet, hands, knees, elbows.
- Difficulty using feet.
- Difficulty sitting for extended periods of time.
- Inability to kneel or squat.
- Pain when moving or lifting the arms or moving the legs.

- Pain when using hands for focused tasks, such as operating scissors, using writing instruments, etc.

What To Do

Schedule an appointment to find out if you are a candidate for the laser therapy at our concierge clinic by calling (888) 716-6028, emailing us at info@ocspinedisc.com, or making an appointment online at www.ocspinedisc.com.

At the Lasermed Institute, we combine the Lifelite Laser Healing System™ with the Graston Technique to treat your symptoms. This process reduces overall muscle, joint, and tendon inflammation. Laser therapy works with, and magnifies, your body's natural processes to relieve all types of arthritis pain. Rheumatoid, osteoarthritis, and degenerative diseases that result from spinal osteoarthritis are all treatable in our clinic. We have successfully used laser light to reduce swelling and inflammation by massively increasing blood flow and circulation to the affected areas. The laser technology repairs chemical damage to cells so that they re-energize themselves and begin healing. New collagen is formed, which is the primary support structure of ligaments, tendons, and muscles.

Coupling the laser treatments with the Graston Technique doubles and triples the effects of just using the laser alone. Where the laser is a photonic treatment, the GT is a mechanical treatment. It works to break up the buildup of scar tissue in the affected areas, which unbinds the tendons and joints and gives you greater mobility.

Although we use other forms of therapy at our clinic for a more holistic approach to the management of this disease, the laser process alone may greatly improve the quality of your life in regards to pain relief and activities of daily living. Basic, daily functional activities like walking, sleeping, and exercising can be a part of your life again.

There is no cure for arthritis, but the laser technology is an effective tool for successful management. You will experience an improved quality of life as you are able to conquer the pain and inflammation that conquered you for so long.

Case Study

"Now I can get up without that excruciating pain in my knee."
<u>Arthritic Knees</u>

"I came in to see Dr. Phillip because I had pain in my knees. I previously had tried Cortisol shots, and that was temporary relief – 3 to 4 months. I saw an ad in the LA Times, so I decided to give Dr. Phillip a call. Today is my third day of laser treatment and now I can get up and stand up without that excruciating pain in my knee."

Cheryl Welch, Corona, CA

(You can see Cheryl's review by typing "Cheryl's Lifelite Laser Arthritic Knee Pain Cure" into the YouTube.com search bar.)

Chapter 13

Fibromyalgia Syndrome

Fibromyalgia is one of the most common musculoskeletal health problems, but can be hard to diagnose in the world of medicine. It is not uncommon for those who suffer to go to a wide range of doctors, only to be told that their illness is in their head. It's no wonder that this syndrome often leads to depression and social isolation.

This is an illness that affects the whole body, and interferes with the quality of life on a day-to-day basis. Those who suffer long term are extremely exhausted, but ironically have sleep problems. Often, there is only enough energy to lie on the couch, watching the seasons of life pass by. It can be lonely, discouraging, painful, and depressing.

What It Is

By definition, a syndrome is a set of symptoms. Fibromyalgia syndrome is a chronic health problem that causes widespread pain and tenderness throughout the body – to the point where you are sensitive to the touch. The pain is not central to one location, and can in fact move to different areas. Since the pain can come and go - and move - this makes misdiagnosis easy and frequent. There is no traditional test to detect fibromyalgia, and it is often diagnosed only after expensive lab tests or X-rays have been able to rule out a wide range of other possibilities.

Identifying the Onset and Symptoms

Although there is some speculation on the actual causes of the disease, it is most often triggered by something, like an outside trauma or other illness. This could include things like spinal problems, a car accident, or any number of other diseases and physical stressors. Even emotional stress can induce the onset.

Symptoms of fibromyalgia and other related issues can vary in intensity over time. They do not always get progressively worse, but an improvement today does not mean there will not be a severe flare up later. Stress often increases the severity of the symptoms. Ironically, the syndrome itself can often bring a greater degree of stress into your life, which can trigger a vicious cycle.

Symptoms include:

- Joint and muscle tenderness to the touch.
- Fatigue
- Sleep problems (waking up groggy).
- Difficulty thinking and problems with memory.

Some patients also may have:

- Depression or anxiety.
- Migraine or tension headaches.
- Digestive problems, including irritable bowel syndrome, or gastro esophageal reflux disease.
- An irritable or overactive bladder.
- Pelvic pain.
- TMJ - a set of symptoms including face or jaw pain, jaw clicking and ringing in the ears.

What To Do

We have successfully treated many patients suffering from Fibromyalgia Syndrome. Women and men who have suffered for years have finally found relief with our cutting edge Lifelite Laser Healing System. The photonic energy helps to heal the physical causes of the disease and bring the body back to its natural, un-agitated state.

Where patients once had little energy and a list of discouraging symptoms, they are now able to take on a more vital lifestyle after only a few treatments. It is so rewarding to see people transform right in front of me, and watch the life come back into their eyes.

In addition to the treatment options available at the Lasermed Pain Institute, there are other things you can do to help offset these heavy symptoms.

- **Take time to relax each day.** You can quickly change your stressed state by using deep-breathing techniques and relaxing your mind through meditation.
- **Commit to a consistent sleep schedule.** Going to bed and waking up at the same time every day can give your body the cues it needs to slip into a better sleeping pattern. As you get the rest you need, you will find that your body is better able to repair itself, both mentally and physically.
- **Avoid Harmful Toxins.** In Southern California, we are surrounded by environmental toxins that are difficult to avoid. But you can certainly control the ones that go in or on your body! Avoiding caffeine, excessive alcohol, smoking, and other chemical toxins can help your body restore itself to health, and better relax when it's time to sleep.
- **Exercise.** Exercise is very important and often helps to reduce pain and fatigue. This may sound counterintuitive, but it is true. As you begin your exercise program, you may need to start slow, as you work through your physical limitations, but sticking with it will help your overall sense of well-being.
- **Schedule a candidacy consultation at our Lasermed Pain Institute:** We use Star Trek-like technology to help ease the burden of your symptoms and go to the root cause behind your fibromyalgia symptoms. Success and rest don't have to wait until tomorrow. Schedule an appointment at our concierge clinic by calling (888) 716-6028, emailing us at dryoo@fixfibromyalgia.com or making an appointment online at www.fixfibromyalgia.com.

Case Study

"I've had lots of different treatments from Mexico to LA, but none of the treatments worked until I came to Dr. Phillip."

Suffering From Fibromyalgia, Arthritis, & Sciatica After a Car Accident

"I've been suffering for 40 years from chronic pain due to a car accident. I've been diagnosed with arthritis, fibromyalgia, and sciatica. I've had lots of different treatments from Mexico to LA, but none of the treatments worked until I came to Dr. Phillip. I was really depressed when I first came here because I had tried almost everything and it all failed. But lo and behold, the treatments did work, and I'm feeling a lot better! I've been coming twice a week at the Lasermed Pain Institute, and Dr. Phillip has been taking very good care of me. He's been extremely patient, and has given me many treatments so I'm very happy. For those people out there who are really, really suffering you can go anywhere you like and check everything out, but you'd be very crazy not to come to Dr. Yoo first. So please pick up the phone and call now!"

Patricia Voss, Costa Mesa, CA

(You can see Patricia's amazing testimonial by typing "Patricia's fibromyalgia laser" into the YouTube.com search bar.)

Chapter 14

Peripheral Neuropathy

I can especially empathize with those of you suffering from neuropathy, a condition that affects the nerves spreading through your body. That's because this is something that I have suffered through four different times in my life. I understand the confusion and hopelessness that can come after consulting with a physician, who will tell you that there is nothing that can be done and that you just have to get used to living this way.

Most people associate neuropathy with diabetes and aging bodies. I definitely broke that mold in every way possible. My worst case of neuropathy was a result of an injury I sustained while lifting weights during the prime of my life. I was doing an exercise called the front squat, where you have one big bar in your hand. I was holding too much weight and the bar was pressing its weight into my fingertip, which caused numbness, tingling, and needle-like pains.

Normally, those kinds of sensations will go away following a workout, but this time they didn't. I developed such severe numbness and pins and needle-like pain that I couldn't even type. It affected me every day. I was aware of it while on the computer, brushing my teeth, preparing a meal – it was always in the way.

Part of me believed the doctor – that there was no hope and no cure. That part of me lost hope. Then there was the other part of me that refused to give up looking. That was the part that had pushed me to travel the world looking for solutions to the body's problems. I'm happy to say that was the part of me that won.

What It Is

Peripheral Neuropathy is a term used to describe any nerve disorder outside of the brain. In Latin, "Peripheral" means any part of your body below your head, "Neuro" means nerve, and "Pathy" means disease. Furthermore, the term neuropathy refers to the nerve damage caused by various conditions such as diabetes, chemotherapy, infections, and vitamin deficiencies (you can see the longer list below). When a nerve is damaged, it can affect any area of the body since it acts as a highway from the brain to the rest of your body to deliver information. Any area of the body can be affected by neuropathy. The affected area could include the joints, muscles, internal organs, skin, or a combination of these areas of the body.

Causes

One of the most common causes of neuropathy is diabetes. Half of the people diagnosed with diabetes will also suffer from neuropathy. In that case, it will be referred to as diabetic neuropathy. Although it can affect any of the nerves in the body, diabetic neuropathy typically affects the nerves in the hands and feet most severely.

There are a number of other causes of neuropathy as well. These include the following:

- Chemotherapy
- Cholesterol medication (statin drugs)
- Side effects from other medications
- Spinal stenosis
- Herniated Discs
- Degenerative Disc Disease
- Alcoholism
- Exposure to some types of toxins or other kinds of poisons
- Contact with a pesticide, black mold, or other neurotoxin
- Environmental toxins in the work place or home
- Too much aspartame (neurotoxin), as in diet colas or other sugar-free products
- Infections
- Genetic disorders
- Tumors that exert pressure on the surrounding nerves
- Trauma to the nerve, like from an auto accident or other injury
- Extended pressure on the nerve

- Repetitive movements such as typing, which can also lead to Carpal Tunnel Syndrome
- Autoimmune diseases, like rheumatoid arthritis and lupus

Different Types of Neuropathy

Peripheral neuropathy tends to be used by physicians as an umbrella term for all types of neuropathy, but there have been more than one hundred types of neuropathy categorized so far. The following are just a few of the more than one hundred types of neuropathy:

- **Peripheral Neuropathy** is termed as nerve damage that is located in the nerves that are on the outside of the main nerves. Peripheral Neuropathy damages nerves in your feet, legs, arms and hands. Peripheral neuropathy is also called sensory neuropathy and generally affects the feet and legs with the most severity. It produces muscle weakness and loss of reflexes, especially at the ankle, leading to changes in walking. Foot deformities may develop such as hammertoes and the arch may collapse. Blisters and sores may start to appear on numb foot areas due to unnoticed pressure or injury. These injuries can develop infections, which may spread to the bone and result in amputation. It is estimated that half of amputations are preventable if these kinds of issues are identified and treated in time.
- **Diabetic Neuropathy** is a frequent side effect seen in people who have diabetes. It is typically characterized by numbness, pain and tingling in the hands and feet. In more severe cases, complications can be seen in other bodily systems as well. These include the kidneys, urinary tract, heart, digestive system, and blood vessels.
- **Cranial Neuropathy** affects the nerves that are joined at the brain. These nerves control the sensations of taste, hearing, and sight. As a result, there are often many complications of the eye.
- **Charcot's Joint**, or neuropathic arthropathy, affects the stability of the joints. This type of neuropathy frequently affects the feet, which can eventually result in the inability to walk.
- **Autonomic Neuropathy** affects the nerves of the heart, affecting blood pressure and blood glucose levels. It also affects

internal organs, causing problems with digestion, respiratory function, urination, sexual response, and vision. Difficulty controlling urination, frequent urinary tract infections, erectile dysfunction, and digestion issues are most commonly found in this type of neuropathy.

Identifying Onset and Symptoms

Depending on the type of your neuropathy, there can be a wide range of pains, numbness and side effects. Although neuropathy can affect any part of the body, it most commonly affects the extremities - the hands and feet. Many forms of neuropathy begin in the feet before moving onward throughout the rest of the body.

Left untreated, there is typically a progressive worsening of the condition. Similarly, the most common organ that is affected by neuropathy is the skin. Typically, the condition progresses from the outside in, with the skin being affected first, then the internal organs eventually being affected if the neuropathy is allowed to continue its progression unabated. Usually neuropathy is a slow moving, yet progressive condition. There are some types of neuropathy, however, that progress at a much quicker pace. Fortunately, with the proper treatment implemented as quickly as possible, the effects of almost all types of neuropathy can be significantly slowed.

Symptoms include:

- Burning, tingling, loss of sensitivity and numbness in the hands and/or feet
- Sharp pains and cramps
- Loss of balance or coordination
- Sensitivity to touch, even light touching
- Shaking and lightheadedness
- High heart rate
- Severe pain in pelvis, eyes, chest, shins, abdomen
- Bell's Palsy on one side of the face
- Clumsiness and weakness when moving
- Weak bladder
- Burning, tingling, loss of sensitivity and numbness in the hands and/or feet
- Dizziness when standing
- . Unable to feel textures or temperatures

- Erectile dysfunction
- Infections
- Double vision

What To Do

Unfortunately, there is a point in neuropathy where the damage is so extensive that our "no drug, no surgery" approach can no longer be effective. This means that the sooner we examine the extent of your nerve damage, the better. So before your nerve damage becomes more severe, irreversible, or permanent I encourage you to find out if you are a candidate for the Lifelite Laser Neuropathy Elimination Program by contacting our Lasermed Neuropathy Institute by calling (888) 716-6028, emailing us at dryoo@lasermedinstitute.com, or making an appointment online at www.noneuropathy.com.

I have found that a combination of a variety of treatments centered on the world's most powerful Class IV Lifelite Laser is the solution to most cases of neuropathy. I am speaking on my own behalf, as well as the long list of patients that I have successfully treated for this. I used this therapy four times with stellar results. This means that I am able to stand as my own testimonial for this powerful therapy.

Our patented and unique Lifelite Lasers put out 60-250 watts of continuous or super-pulsed photonic energy, which is five to 30 times more powerful than all the other lasers out there; most Class IV lasers put out between 7.5 to15 watts of photonic energy. Our laser penetrates deeper into the tissues to bring you superior and faster clinical results. The blast of photonic energy increases the circulation by increasing nitric oxide production to open up the blood vessels. This enables your body to better pump its life-giving blood supply to all areas of the body, including those negatively affected by neuropathy. Furthermore, the photobiostimulation from the laser stimulates stem cells to help regenerate the worn out protective covering of the nerve called the myelin sheath. In fact, most neuropathies are caused by the wear and tear, or stripping off of the protective sheath, exposing the nerve fibers to damage and dysfunction.

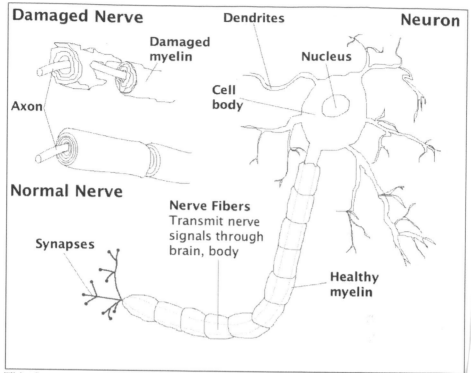

This figure shows how damaged myelin sheath (the protective covering of nerves) causes a disruption in the nerve's ability to transmit normal signals throughout the body, causing neuropathic pain, numbness, weakness, etc. Our Lifelite Laser stimulates the repair of the damaged nerve tissue, which alleviates peripheral neuropathy symptoms.

Most of our patients suffering from neuropathy have tried other forms of treatment with little to no relief. Our cutting-edge, futuristic technologies enable us to provide relief to 90.1% of our patients.

The majority of patients will see the best results from the combination of the laser treatment and natural food supplements. This approach allows the body to heal itself naturally from the inside, as well as the outside. In our clinic, we offer the Neuropathy Support Formula, which uses vitamins and anti-oxidants to lesson and prevent the flare up of painful symptoms.

The Neuropathy Support Formula is a combination of the following natural ingredients:

- B1 Vitamins – can help the effects of neuropathy, general nerve damage, as well as the overall health of a diabetic's coronary and improve the health of those that are not diabetic.
- B12 Vitamin – has been said, by clinical studies, to redevelop nerves. B12 can also increase the protein in your body, which ultimately helps in giving life back to your nerves.
- Alpha-Lipoic acid – helps to get the blood moving and oxidants to be released, providing oxygen to make its way to damaged nerves, which ease the pain of neuropathy in feet and hands.
- Propriety Blend – assists in balancing a person's blood sugar levels, restores strength to a weakened nervous system and gives pain relief to the damaged nerve cells.

Case Studies

"My son-in-law and my daughter were firm believers in what the laser had done for my legs after just one treatment."

Diabetic Neuropathy & Severe Edema

"I've been a neuropathy patient for about 10 years, but when I met Dr. Yoo my life changed. He didn't think he could do anything for me at first, but he told me that he'd give me three treatments and let me know whether or not he could help me. So right there I was impressed by the doctor. My son-in-law, an administrative coordinator at Kaiser, on the other hand was a huge skeptic. Dr. Yoo decided to come to the old folk's home to meet with my son-in-law and my daughter, a physical therapist at Kaiser for about 28 years. After they spoke to each other, my son-in-law and my daughter were firm believers in what the laser had done for my legs, especially after they took a look at my legs after just one treatment. Even my own home health care doctor was impressed by the change and wanted to speak to Dr. Yoo immediately. Everybody that I've spoken to and have seen my legs were extremely impressed and couldn't believe it. It's been a terrific change and I owe it all to Dr. Yoo for everything he's done for me."

Walter Cox, Korean War Veteran, Cerritos, CA

(You can see Walter's incredible transformation by typing "Walter's Diabetic Neuropathy Laser" into the YouTube.com search bar.)

"I noticed a very big difference after one visit."

<u>Non Diabetic, Idiopathic Neuropathy</u>

"I am a retired Plastic and Reconstructive surgeon in Santa Ana. In the last 5 years, I have developed neuropathy and fortunately I am not a diabetic so I'm glad it's idiopathic. The pain was so bad all day and night that I hoped it did not come to them amputating my feet eventually. I have taken all kinds medications you could think of and nothing has worked. Finally, I read in the papers about Dr. Yoo who had a LRX 60 watt laser instead of the 12 watt laser like what most doctors have. I went to another doctor and it did not do me any good because I still had the pain day and night. In any case, after one visit with Dr. Yoo and his LRX 60 laser I noticed a very big difference after one visit. My pain went from a 10 down to a 5 and that is for both pain and numbness. I have gotten to almost feeling the floor again with my feet. My neuropathy is getting better and better and I hope to one day very soon be able to run around the block how I use to. Thanks to the good care of Dr. Yoo and his staff."

Joseph Cavon, M.D., Santa Ana, CA

(You can see Dr. Joe's raving review by typing "Dr. Cavon's Neuropathy Laser" into the YouTube.com search bar.)

"The prickling pains in my feet are less and I can start walking again without my wife's help!!"

<u>Neuropathy with Prickling Pain & Short Steps</u>

"I'm a retired general surgeon from Laguna Niguel. I'm in pretty good health except for my neuropathy. I came to know about Dr. Yoo by publications in newspaper. I was very bothered by prickling pain in my feet, my steps were shorter, and I also noticed a change in my sense of balance. Although I have seen similar doctors in the past, I decided to see Dr. Yoo because he combined therapies. Since I've started the

treatments I believe I have improved very much. My pain has definitely decreased, but I'd really appreciate it if Dr. Yoo can eventually help me with my walking, because I'm not used to taking these short steps. Yet, I have improved nonetheless because I'm now starting to walk indoors without the assistance of my wife. I believe these treatments have helped me, and I hope that if I continue my treatments I will also be better at walking. I'd be extremely grateful to Dr. Yoo if I can eventually get back to walking normally."

Dr. Gumer Garcia, Laguna Niguel, CA

(See the doctor's transformation by typing "Dr. Garcia's food numbness & tingling laser" into the YouTube.com search bar.)

"After only my first treatment, the immense tingling in my feet had subsided."

Peripheral Neuropathy with Loss Of Balance

"I'm a retired nurse from Fullerton, CA. I was diagnosed 10 years ago with peripheral neuropathy. I had come into Orange County Laser Spine and Neuropathy Center recommended by my physical therapist, who had told me that Class IV lasers were the only thing that he had seen that worked for peripheral neuropathy. After only my first treatment, the immense tingling in my feet had subsided. After the second treatment, I was able to drive myself for the first time in two months! I have to just thank Dr. Yoo and the staff profusely for all they're doing for me."

Sharon Orabona, R.N. Fullerton, CA

(You can see Sharon's amazing testimonial by typing "Sharon's Laser Neuropathy" into the YouTube.com search bar.)

"I've had three laser treatments now and the tingling is all gone!"

Neuropathy From Chemotherapy & Shoulder Injury

"I had chemotherapy twice from cancer, which left me with tingling in my feet, and they were so numb they felt like needles poking through

them. I've had three laser treatments now and the tingling is all gone. They're still a little bit numb, but the major thing I came in here for was a bad shoulder. I couldn't raise my arm but 45 degrees and after the third treatment I can raise it all the way up over my head with no problem at all! I play handball, so you can imagine what it means to me. I thank Dr. Yoo for treating me as good as he has."

Jim Carson, San Clemente, CA

(You can see Jim's amazing transformation by typing "Jim Can Laser" into the YouTube.com search bar.)

Chapter 15

Neuralgia (Nerve Pains)
(See also Neuropathy)

I once had an older patient, a former professor at California Polytechnic, come to my office who had been suffering from shingles and neuralgia for over 10 years and had "tried everything under the sun" to relieve his pain. My heart went out to him as he told me his story, and how he'd been in pain 24 hours a day for over a decade.

I think back over the things I've done in the last 10 years – travelling to different countries, evolving my practice, serving my community – and compare that with the last 10 years of his, as he maintained a spectator position in his own life. Imagine going from that to living pain free. Imagine all the things you would do with such a sudden invitation to live again.

In some small way, I can understand what he was going through, as I suffered my own bout of severe shingles. For me, it attacked my lumbar nerve, which branches off your low back, down your gluteus all the way to your hamstring, down the side of your leg and even into your groin. I still have the scars from the blistering.

Shingles was one of the things that I first sought laser treatment for myself – the same treatment I am successfully using in my practice today.

What It Is

Neuralgia is a sharp, lighting bolt of pain that extends through the path of a nerve. It is caused by irritation to or damage of a nerve. It is considered to be a type of neuropathy. The most common neuralgias include postherpetic neuralgia (shingles) and trigeminal neuralgia.

Identifying Onset and Symptoms

In many instances, the cause of neuralgia is unknown. Shingles is a derivative of the Chicken Pox virus, and is most likely to flare when your immune system is weak. When you get shingles, you want to treat it as fast as you can, or you run the risk of getting permanent nerve damage. The scar tissue can accumulate on the nerve, which can cause permanent numbness, pain, and damage to the nerve.

Symptoms include:

- Increased sensitivity of the skin along the length of the damaged nerve. Any amount of touch or pressure induces pain.
- Numbness along the nerve path.
- A sharp, stabbing pain. This may come and go, or be constant.
- Weakness or paralysis of muscles that are fed by the affected nerve.
- You may stop sweating, since nerves control this function.

Causes

- Chemical irritation.
- Diabetes
- Infections, such as shingles, Lyme disease and syphilis.
- Side effects of some medications.
- Pressure being put on the nerve by nearby bones, ligaments, blood vessels or tumors.
- Injury and trauma, including surgery.

What To Do

Find out if you are a candidate for laser therapy by calling our concierge clinic at (888) 716-6028, or emailing us at info@ocspinedisc.com.

There are a lot of treatments suggested by doctors, some of which can make the problem worse by either increasing the pain or totally deadening the treated area. Often, this condition is misdiagnosed, which prolongs the time it takes for a proper diagnosis.

In our clinic, we use The Lifelite Laser Healing System to address the issue. We have done this with stunning success. Patients who have suffered debilitating pain for an extended period of time find relief and are able to go back to living again.

Case Studies

"The laser gave me enormous relief from the itching of the shingles."

<u>Shingles & Extreme Itching</u>

"I have suffered with shingles for three and a half years. I have tried acupuncture, all forms of pills, and all sorts of remedies. I found Dr. Yoo's ad in the L.A. Times of the laser treatment for my shingles, so I thought I would come and give it a try. The first three treatments I got with the laser gave me enormous relief from the itching of the shingles because it drove me crazy for years. They come and go, but now that I have had several treatments I feel a 60% improvement or maybe even more. I am very pleased with the results that have occurred with my treatments. I look forward for my maintenance program. Thank you Dr. Yoo."

Joe Muniz, Costa Mesa, CA

(You can see Patricia's Joe's amazing transformation by typing "Joe's neuralgia shingles laser" into the YouTube.com search bar.)

"I believe that I am 100% cured."

<u>Neuralgia & Jaw Pain</u>

"Since September of 2010 I have suffered from excruciating pain on my jaw line from one side to the other. I have been to regular doctors, as well as neurologists. I was diagnosed with neuralgia and they put me on Neurontin starting at 100mg then increasing it to 800mg. Still I was suffering. After visiting Dr. Phillip Yoo he suggested one laser treatment as a trial and within minutes I could feel a huge difference. Now I am only down to 300mg of the medication. After this week I

will be cutting the medication to 100mg. I believe that I am 100% cured. Thank you Dr. Yoo."

Linda Hodge, Orange, CA

(You can see Linda's miracle by typing "Linda's Jaw Laser Neuropathy" into the YouTube.com search bar.)

Chapter 16

Carpal Tunnel Syndrome

When you're living with carpal tunnel syndrome, even small daily tasks can be daunting and full of pain. I know because I have lived with it. This condition is usually caused by repetitive stresses. For me, my downfall was my passion for working out; I probably tweaked my wrist one too many times in the gym.

Carpal Tunnel Syndrome affects the wrist and hands, which are part of almost everything you do. Typing a quick email, pouring a glass of water, and walking the dog suddenly feel like insurmountable chores. However there is hope – the restoration of 89% of the mobility in my wrist proves it.

What It Is

Carpal Tunnel Syndrome is a disorder that puts pressure on the median nerve, which is the nerve in the wrist supplying feeling and movement to parts of the hand. The median nerve tunnel is normally narrow, so any swelling can pinch the nerve, causing pain, numbness, tingling sensations, or weakness. The condition occurs most often in individuals between the ages of 30 and 60, and is more prevalent in women than in men.

The syndrome is often associated with excessive activities that target the hand and wrist areas, such as writing, typing, driving, etc. But it is also connected to other kinds of health issues.

Medical problems associated with carpal tunnel include:

- Bone fractures and arthritis in the wrist
- Acromegaly

- Diabetes
- Hypothyroidism
- Kidney failure
- Menopause or premenstrual syndrome (PMS)
- Systemic lupus erythematosus (SLE)

Identifying Onset and Symptoms

You will notice some or all of the following symptoms during and after onset:

- Numbness/tingling/weakness in the thumb and next two or three fingers of one or both hands.
- Numbness or tingling in the palm of the hand.
- Pain extending to the elbow.
- Pain in the wrist or hand in one or both hands.
- Problems with fine finger movements (coordination) in one or both hands.
- Wasting away of the muscle under the thumb (in advanced or long-term cases).
- Weak grip or difficulty carrying bags (a common complaint).

What To Do

Some doctors will suggest using a splint for support, medications for pain relief and to reduce inflammation, corticosteroid injections, and even surgery. Those who have desperately resorted to surgery have often reported little to no improvement in their condition.

At the Lasermed Pain Institute, we aim to go to the root of the problem instead of just treating and masking the symptoms. Our cutting edge, non-invasive technology includes no risk factors. We combine the laser therapy with the Graston Technique for maximum results. Coupling the laser treatments with the Graston Technique doubles and triples the effects of just using the laser alone. Where the laser is a photonic treatment, the GT is a mechanical treatment. It works to break up the buildup of scar tissue in the affected areas, which unbinds the tendons and joints and gives you greater mobility.

The laser is placed in contact with the skin, allowing the photon energy to penetrate deep into the tunnel and tissue. The process allows the blood to stimulate the blood supply and improves micro circulation that will increase the amount of cellular nutrition resulting in reduction of inflammation, and expanding the median nerve tunnel in your wrists. Normal cell functions are then restored; these are the results of tissue regeneration and cellular reproduction.

Find out if you are a candidate for our procedures by scheduling an appointment at our concierge clinic by calling (888) 716-6028, emailing us at dryoo@lasermedinstitute.com, or making an appointment online at www.lasermedinstitute.com.

Case Studies

"I don't have to wear wrist braces anymore! These treatments will give you relief, and I believe it is curative."

Carpal Tunnel Syndrome

"I have been under the care of chiropractors since the age of 15, so that would be 43 years! I have always found chiropractic care to help because I have degenerative disc disease on my right side. I have also had issues with sciatica my whole life. I am always looking for new treatments. One day, as I was reading the Orange County Register, *I came across Dr. Phillip Yoo's ad on lumbar decompression laser treatment. I tried lumbar decompression twice in the last year and it gave me great relief. Hearing that Dr. Yoo combined the decompression and laser, I thought that it should give me even more relief and it has been working very well. In addition to my lumbar problems, I had also developed Carpal Tunnel. Dr. Yoo used the Graston method along with the laser to relieve a tremendous amount of pain and after eight treatments, it's completely gone. I don't have to war wrist braces anymore! It is just like everything else; you have to be consistent with it. As long as you keep coming to your appointments, I find that these treatments will give you relief and I believe it is curative. I am extremely happy and very impressed!"*

Lee Pearlman, Newport Coast, CA

(You can Lee's transformation by typing "Lee's Carpal Tunnel" into the YouTube.com search bar.)

"It was the most relief I'd ever gotten from a treatment. It was fairly miraculous."

<u>Dupuytren's Contracture & Carpal Tunnel Syndrome</u>

"I have arthritis in my wrist and hands. I just thought there was nothing I could do with it. I can't take pain pills because it affects my kidneys, so I was stuck with chronic pain. My pain wasn't extreme, but it was a nuisance constantly — at about a five or six [on the pain scale]. I tried everything — heat, cold, injections, and pain meds over the years. I felt excellent after the first treatment. It was the most relief I'd ever gotten from a treatment. It was fairly miraculous."

Jay Allen, Retired CIA Agent

(You can see Jay's raving review by typing "Jay's Wrist Miracle Treatment" into the YouTube.com search bar.)

Chapter 17

Sciatica (Leg Pains)

Sciatica is something I thoroughly understand, since this is something that I have suffered from. I remember how frustrating it was not being able to drive without sharp pains shooting through my leg. I was immobilized. On a scale of one to 10, it was a 10. I understand the look of desperation in my patients' eyes as they walk in the door hoping for relief.

I was a practicing chiropractor when my sciatica set in. After travelling the world and picking up the best techniques for pain relief, I was confident that I could solve my problem. However, the tools in my tool box at the time proved to be unequal to the challenge. I was a little embarrassed when I wasn't able to solve my problem; I'd already earned the reputation of the Pain Terminator by then. But the silver lining to my story is that it was actually this condition, combined with some other unbearable conditions and symptoms that got me on the path to discovering the laser technology I use today that gives such powerful results to my patients that suffer from the same issues.

What It Is

The term "Sciatica" can include a number of different resulting conditions all stemming from a root cause. Sciatica is a set of symptoms including pain caused by general compression and/or irritation of one of five spinal nerve roots, or irritation of the left, right, or both sciatic nerves. The pain, tingling, and/or numbness or weakness originates in the lower back and travels through the buttock and down the large sciatic nerve to the back of the leg.

Identifying Onset and Symptoms

Often, a particular event or injury does not cause sciatica, but rather the sciatic nerve pain tends to develop over time. You will notice a burning sensation, numbness, or tingling radiating from the lower back and upper buttock down the back of the thigh to the back of the leg. Sciatica can make daily activities like walking and driving difficult, if not impossible.

Specific sciatica symptoms also vary widely in type, location, and severity, depending upon the condition causing the sciatica. While symptoms can be very painful, it is rare that permanent sciatic nerve damage (tissue damage) will result.

Symptoms include:

- Shooting pain when walking or bending at the waist.
- Sharp stabbing pains when moving the legs in certain positions.
- Numbness in the feet and toes.
- Trouble controlling your limbs.
- Loss of balance.
- Shooting Pains.

What To Do

Contact our concierge clinic by calling (888) 716-6028, emailing us at info@ocspinedisc.com, or making an appointment online at www.ocspinedisc.com, to see if you are a candidate for our The Lifelite Laser Healing System.

This cutting-edge, futuristic technology delivers photonic energy straight to the nerve, where it aids the body in the healing process. The laser therapy works to heal the peripheral components to the problem, too. Often, sciatica is caused by factors like herniated or bulging discs. In those instances, this healing photonic energy actually heals the damaged disc and reverses the problem entirely. This isn't just a system for relieving the symptoms, but for correcting and removing the problem.

Case Studies

"After two laser treatments, I was healed! The sciatica was completely gone and I was able to go ballroom dancing again!"

<u>Painful Sciatica After Pain Killers</u>

"I'm a retired registered nurse from UCLA Medical Center. I had bad sciatica and tried everything including painkillers. None of it helped at all. One day, I was reading the newspaper and saw Dr. Yoo's article. I then decided that I would see him. After two laser treatments, I was healed! The sciatica was completely gone. I was able to walk. I was also able to do my ballroom dancing again. Thank you Dr. Yoo! You're the greatest!"

Emmy Beltran, R.N., Los Angeles, CA

(You can see Emmy's raving review by typing "Emmy Sciatic Laser" into the YouTube.com search bar.)

"After just 7 laser treatments, the upper & lower leg pains I have had for 45 years are finally better!"

<u>Sciatica With Pain & Tightness In The Back</u>
<u>Of The Legs, Hips, & Lower Back</u>
<u>After Chiropractic Care</u>

"I've been in severe pain for about six or eight months. The pain goes down the back of both my legs, my hips, and my lower back. I had been going to a chiropractic doctor for years and years. I've had pain in my back for about 45 years off and on in different places and I tried laser last year with another doctor. It took a lot of sessions, but it worked. Then all of sudden the pain started in both of my legs. I saw an ad in the Orange County Register *and I came in initially with my husband because he had neuropathy and I wanted him to try the laser. Dr. Phil ended up examining me as well and I decided to try it on my legs. Today is my seventh treatment and I feel at least 40% better. The pain in my lower legs is much better and the pain in the upper legs is definitely better. I'm not exactly where I want to be so I hope to continue treatment until all the pain is gone."*

Cherry Ellis, Buena Park, CA

(You can see Cherry's amazing testimonial by typing "Cherry's Sciatic Laser" into the YouTube.com search bar.)

Appendix

Common questions
about the world's most powerful
Class IV therapeutic lasers

Q: How did you get so successful in treating those suffering
from the most difficult to treat pain syndromes?

I traveled the world for over 15 years, doing a lot of research with
combining traditional and alternative treatments for those suffering
from severe pain. I first experimented combining phototherapy with
acupuncture while working as a medical missionary in Central America,
and I got decent results. I then ran two pain clinics in Korea where I
treated the U.S. Army, Air Force, Navy Seal, and other Special Forces
Personnel.

I furthered my studies in chiropractic sports medicine in Europe,
where I and was invited to treat Olympic athletes at the 2008 Beijing
Olympics. During that time, I teamed up with the other sports doctors
to combine Eastern and Western medical procedures and got great
results. I also was solicited to treat entertainers on tour such as
Beyoncé and the Pussy Cat Dolls due to the reputation of getting
performers back on stage as soon as possible when injured

After all my research, which spanned four continents, I came to the
conclusion that although the combination of allopathic and alternative
therapies benefited most of the population, there were always those
stubborn cases that did not respond to either drugs, injections, surgery,
or even conservative therapies such as physical therapy, acupuncture,
chiropractic, etc. I knew there had to be something else to offer these

folks suffering from the worst stubborn pain syndromes, and I have found it in hi-powered laser medicine.

After moving to Southern California, my concierge clinic is now servicing Hollywood actors, supermodels, and a multitude of NFL, Major League Baseball, volleyball, and other professional athletes due to the laser's fast healing ability.

It is very rewarding to contribute to getting elite soldiers back on their missions, athletes back to competition, and entertainers and celebrities back on stage in relatively little time.

Q: How did you get into Laser Medicine?

Upon returning to the United States, low and behold, I had injured my back doing vigorous CrossFit exercises, and was diagnosed with a herniated disc and sciatica. The pain was so bad I could not even drive more than 30 minutes without the sharp electrical-like pain shooting down my buttock and leg. Needless to say, I had tried everything from spinal decompression to chiropractic, but nothing relieved it.

Fortunately, I discovered Class IV hi-powered laser therapy. Within a few short weeks, the sciatic pain totally disappeared! Incidentally, I had also suffered from a bad case of shingles, which caused severe peripheral neuropathic pain in my back, buttocks, and groin. I had even developed some neuropathic numbness and tingling in my lateral foot and ankle. Again, it was the laser therapy that saved the day for me.

That herniated disc and neuropathy turned out to be a blessing in disguise, as I had finally discovered the Holy Grail of non-invasive pain management through using hi-powered Class IV laser medicine.

Q: What makes your Class IV laser different from others?

The ability of the laser to deliver sufficient photonic energy in deep tissue is proportionate to the laser's power, and power is measured in watts. Most Class IV lasers only produce six to 12 watts of photonic energy. Our Lifelite 60-watt Hot Laser, and now our Lumix 250-watt super pulsed Cold Laser, deliver five to 33 times more power than any other laser out there. Thus, we get deeper and more powerful healing laser energy into the tissue, resulting in shortened treatment times and superior clinical results.

Q: How many laser sessions are necessary for each patient?

There are typically three stages of hi-powered laser therapy. In phase 1, the main goal is to relieve the pain, inflammation, and numbness. This allows the patient to graduate to phase 2, which involves rehabilitative exercises and deep healing and strengthening of damaged soft tissue, nerves, discs, and bones. Phase 3 is the optimum function phase. This is when your nerve, joint, and soft tissue function is restored, allowing the patient to return to a normal active lifestyle. It is often recommended to get a preventative and maintenance visit with the doctor every few months or so to make sure you stay well.

That being said, although many people note relief after just a handful of sessions, we encourage patients to take advantage of a full treatment course, as each laser exposure builds upon each other, and it often takes some time to allow the tissue to completely heal. A common mistake is for patients to discontinue treatment after their symptoms subside, which often leads to a return of the painful symptoms because they did not complete the rehabilitative and optimum function phases of treatment.

The appropriate number of sessions for each patient's condition will be determined by the physician. Please be aware that other clinics that use low-level laser therapy, particularly with inexpensive handheld devices, are unlikely to produce the same therapeutic results as our hi-powered lasers. To find out if you are a candidate for hi-powered laser therapy, please visit www.lasermedinstitute.com.

Q: Is the Class IV hi-powered laser therapy covered by insurance and Medicare?

When I came back to the U.S. I played the insurance game and billed Medicare and private insurances for our therapies, only to find that they either refused to pay or did not cover the laser procedures at all*. I felt frustrated that the insurance companies and government-run Medicare tied my hands as a doctor and I could not deliver the proper care that my patients desperately needed.

I also recognized that other costly procedures, such as Lasik, dental implants, laser skin care, etc., are not covered by insurances, but people still invest in these valuable services because they realize that you can't put a price on the healthier and higher quality life these procedures provide.

As a result, I stopped relying on the insurance industry, and decided to create the concierge clinic concept, where the patients pay a fair fee to us directly. This allows the patient to get the care they need, and allows me to be able to deliver superior high-quality health care, without the red tape of dealing with insurances. This benefits both parties, as our staff time is 100% devoted to the patient, instead of wasting time and resources fighting the insurance companies, which only leads to patient and practitioner frustration.

It amazes me that people will agree to a very risky $150,000 spinal surgery, and then undergo that same risky procedure again and again when it fails to alleviate their pain and disability, *just because insurance will pay for it*. What is the use of having insurance, if you can't even enjoy a pain free and active lifestyle and retirement? Instead, why not spend just 5% of that to have your back pain treated by non-invasive and FDA-cleared safe procedures like our hi-powered Class IV laser therapy?

You should never let the insurance companies dictate your quality of life. Ultimately, *you* are responsible for taking care of your own health and longevity.

* Insurance benefits are always changing, so it is best that you contact your insurance provider directly to find out if the Class IV laser therapy is covered at all, although I wouldn't count on it.

Q: Can you tell us about any successful cases of patients who have undergone your laser procedure?

Dr. Renaldo Landero, M.D., a famous Geriatric Specialist from Carson, came in with severe neck and neuropathic arm pain from degenerated discs in his cervical spine. His pain was significantly reduced after only a few hi-powered laser treatments.

NFL Player David Jones (also known as DJ), former Offensive Tackle for the Baltimore Ravens and Philadelphia Eagles, came to my office with a bulging disc, a bad case of sciatica, and damaged ankles and feet – obviously all football injuries. He couldn't even drive without a painful flare-up, so you can imagine how this was affecting his game. He flew in from the East Coast in order to get access to my Lifelite

Laser Healing System, and we've seen dramatic results. We took his number on the pain scale down from an eight, all the way to a one or two.

Carla Visnic, a registered nurse, came in with crippling peripheral neuropathy pain and tingling in her feet for over 20 years. She'd been taking Lyrica, Cymbalta, and Gabapentin with no relief. After just three treatments with the 60-watt laser, her pain scale dropped from a 10 to a six, and she got feeling back in her feet.

Q: Can laser therapy help everyone?

NO. Unfortunately, the laser cannot help in all cases. There is a point with some chronic pain, spine, and neuropathy conditions where the damage is so extensive that NO DRUG, NO SURGERY – not even the laser approach – can be effective. So the sooner we examine the extent and severity of your health condition, the better. We use these very specific protocols that help to regenerate damaged nerves, helping nerves to function better. This helps to decrease pain and reduce the other symptoms associated with a diagnosis of spinal, disc, myalgia, and peripheral neuropathy. We are using very specific, state of the art, breakthrough, non-invasive and non-drug treatment procedures for the relief of severe and constant back, joint, foot, and leg pains caused by nerve disorders.

Q: How available is the Class IV 60-watt and 250-watt hi-powered laser procedure to those suffering from chronic pain?

The problem is that because we are the only 60-watt Class IV laser provider on the entire West Coast, we have no choice but to limit the amount of cases we take. If we take too many, the quality of our care would drop, and we refuse to compromise our 5-star quality of care standards.

So to make the Lrx60K hi-powered laser available to more chronic pain sufferers, I am starting a Laser Medicine University where I will be training other doctors on our state-of-the-art laser medicine protocols, and how to implement the client centered, concierge clinic concept.

Q: How does the laser work to treat degenerative discs, spinal stenosis, peripheral neuropathies, and fibromyalgia?

To keep it simple, the laser increases the healing response by delivering photonic energy to damaged discs, soft tissue, and nerves through a process called photobiomodulation. ATP, Oxygen, and blood are delivered to damaged tissue, which decreases inflammation and speeds circulation and healing. Just as sunlight stimulates vegetation to grow through photosynthesis, or produces vitamin D3 when it is absorbed to make strong bones, there is strong evidence that the laser energy stimulates stem cells to regenerate damaged disc, nerve, joint, and soft tissue injuries.

Q: What other conditions can be treated with the hi-powered 60-watt continuous beam and 250-watt super-pulsed beam lasers?

We have had excellent results with treating those suffering from fibromyalgia, carpal tunnel, shingles postherpatic neuralgia, golfer's/tennis elbow, tendinitis and tendinosis of the shoulder, and a host of other nerve, joint, muscular, inflammatory and degenerative disorders.

Please keep in mind that like any medical procedure, the laser is not a cure-all and we often refer or co-manage difficult cases with other medical professionals. In fact, we often refer and co-manage patients between Hoag Hospital, Kaiser Permanente, UCI Medical Center, and other specialists. This ensures that our patients can have access to the best doctors around.

(To see the world's most powerful Class IV laser in action, type "World's most powerful 250 watt super pulsed laser spinal stenosis neuropathy treatment" into the YouTube.com search bar.)

Q: What should chronic sufferers do?

If you or someone you know has a sport, spine, neuropathy, or other chronic pain disorder, first contact your primary care medical provider to rule out any severe underlying conditions. If you have already been to other specialists and you are still suffering, then contact us today at (888) 716-6028 to find out if you are a candidate for the hi-powered laser pain and neuropathy elimination proprietary procedure.

You may also request a free "21st Century Pain Relief Secrets" information package and DVD* to be mailed to you now by calling our toll free, hassle free, 24-hour pre-recorded message pain relief hotline at: (888) 682-5350, or by visiting our special information request website at www.lasermedinstitute.com.

For an appointment to see if you are a candidate for the hi-powered laser therapy, call our concierge clinic at (888) 716-6028** or go to www.theconciergeclinic.com.

Limited quantities available so you are encouraged to order yours today.

** *Mention the "21st Century Pain Relief Book", reader code 21CM, and get a special VIP reader's rate applied on your first consultation with Dr. Yoo to find out if you are a candidate for his proprietary pain relieving Lifelite Laser Healing System. Limited appointments are available. You are encouraged to call now before your condition gets worse and potentially irreversible, or being put on a long waiting list; patients from all over the U.S. and many other countries fly in to see Dr. Yoo, so he is typically booked about one month in advance.*

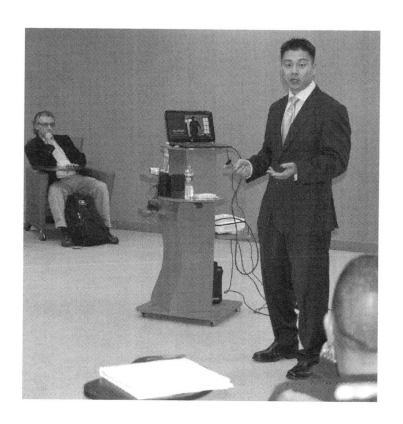

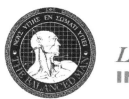 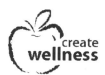

Dr. Phil is a sought after motivational speaker and is ideal for speaking events on the most up to date trends in pain management, weight loss, functional medicine, nutrition, fitness, self-improvement, and how to lead a balanced, spiritual, and healthy lifestyle.

www.lasermedinstitute.com

1 (888) 716-6028